ALL MY FRIENDS ARE CRAZY

I0104199

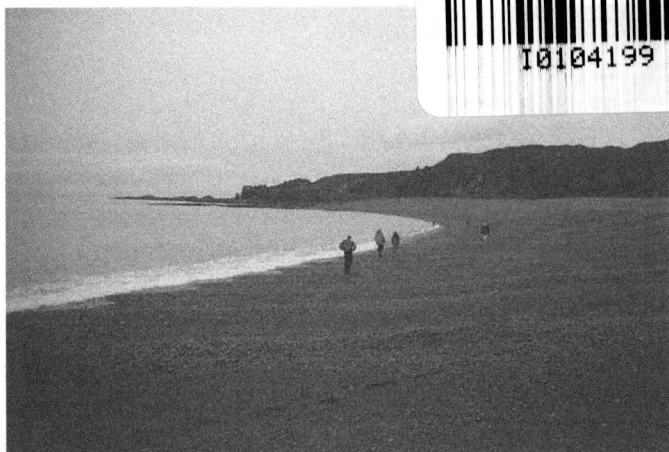

BY SERA ANSTADT
Translated by Sarah Lawson

'One million people commit suicide every year.'
The World Health Organization

SERA ANSTADT

Published by
Chipmunkapublishing
PO Box 6872
Brentwood
Essex CM13 1ZT
United Kingdom

http://www.chipmunkapublishing.co.uk

Translation copyright © Sarah Lawson 2007

Originally published in The Netherlands
as *Al mijn vrienden zijn gek: de dagen van een schizofrene jongen* by BZZToH in Den Haag in 1983

Title page photo by Sarah Lawson

Cover picture: *Guitar study* by Sarah Lawson

Proof-read by Anna Gomez

Translator's Note

Sera Anstadt's touching story of her son's schizophrenia was published in Holland in 1983 and soon went through numerous reprintings and became a minor classic. The story itself begins in the mid-1960s, when Raf (short for Rafael) Keller was a teenager. At first Sera Anstadt could not understand what was wrong with her son, whose behaviour gradually went from sensitive to eccentric to strange to psychotic. She found that social workers and the medical profession were startlingly unhelpful just when she needed all the support she could get. The theories of R.D. Laing were in the ascendancy then: "It became increasingly clear to me how inhumanely social workers could behave because they believed in a new theory," Anstadt says.

In the years covered by this memoir Raf is in various psychiatric institutions as well as at home being cared for by his mother. He is given medication, sometimes, apparently, on an experimental basis. Over the years his mother goes from hope to despair and back again. Along the way she meets some health-care professionals who offer sensitive understanding and others who are cruel and offensive.

We learn to understand the reactions of Sera Anstadt and share her mystification at what is happening to her son. Through his mother we also become acquainted with Raf. He is an intelligent boy with a gift for music and friendship.

3

He plays his guitar and dreams of starting a band and going to a conservatory of music. Because of our knowledge of the pair, Raf's descents into psychosis and his mother's attempts at coping are all the more harrowing for the reader.

In the story that follows, Sera Anstadt and her son and daughter Sabina live in Amsterdam. Her ex-husband, Hans Keller, lives in The Hague on the North Sea coast. This text is faithful to the original Dutch, but I have omitted two pages at the end of chapter 10 consisting of a facsimile of a report issued by the Zürich Police when Raf was arrested in Switzerland. It is interesting but adds nothing to the narrative.

Sera Anstadt (b. 1923) has written several other books, including autobiographical novels. She was born in Lvov (formerly in Poland) and recounts in *Een eigen plek* (A Place of One's Own) her family's arrival in Holland in 1930 and her survival of the war under the Occupation. She still lives in Amsterdam.

Raf is now in his mid-50s and lives in a psychiatric institution near Delft. He moves freely about the city and is acquainted with other "street people" there and still sees his family from time to time.

Schizophrenia has never been long out of the news since Raf's earlier days. At the time of writing in 2006, there has just been a news item concerning the redefinition of schizophrenia: the concept should be abolished, according to mental health experts in Britain "because it is a catch-all term which does not define a specific illness and carries a stigma that destroys people's lives". Professor Richard Bentall of the School of Psychological Sciences at the University of Manchester says, "Patients will do better if doctors focus on their symptoms rather than trying to place them in a disease category." The same report continues, "Although the National Institute for Clinical Excellence recommends talking therapies should be tried, most patients are given only heavy-duty drugs" (*The Guardian*, 10 October 2006). The controversies and conflicting advice that Sera Anstadt found 30 years ago in The Netherlands are still present and still provoking discussion in Great Britain now.

Sarah Lawson
London

SERA ANSTADT

Contents

Chapter 1   Worms

Raf is now 30 years old, a withdrawn, seriously disturbed young man who sometimes thinks about the past with a melancholy smile.

Until he was 15 he was cheerful and easy-going, although he could also be troublesome and now and then even strikingly hot tempered. He was good looking: tall with curly black hair, big dark eyes, and broad shoulders. If he was told something he could listen with great concentration, as though he wanted to feel just what the other person felt.

He went in for sports, especially tennis and athletics, and was bright and popular. Many of his friends played an instrument, and he wanted to study musicology. In his room, which was next to mine and which, until the onset of his illness, he had arranged himself, a bed stood against one of the walls; opposite that there was a big desk and next to it a record player and a music stand. Among all his other pursuits, Raf played guitar and liked having his friends in after school to play music. Sabina, my daughter, who was almost two years older, lived on the top floor.

When Raf was three years old I got divorced. In the beginning that was a great shock for him and Sabina, as it probably is for most children who stop seeing their father every day. Raf, especially, often looked at me with big surprised eyes but was too small to understand an explanation and seldom asked directly about Hans, his father. The relationship between Hans, me, and the children

9

became relatively good again quite soon after the divorce. Hans remarried soon afterwards and while the children were still small they stayed with him regularly.

In the beginning Raf often cried quietly in his bed after such a visit at the weekend. I remember once going to tuck him in and seeing his tears. "Raf, why are you crying?"

"I'm not crying," he replied.

"But I can see that you're sad."

He turned away from me. "No," he said and shook his head violently.

I got the impression that he was trying to be brave. I couldn't get him to talk about his sadness, and even then I already had the feeling that he wanted to spare me his troubles.

Sabina was better at controlling her emotions and could talk about them more easily. She protected Raf. The children got along well and were almost always together. Sabina often said later that she had pleasant memories of her childhood. A nice harmony prevailed among us. Raf and Sabina eventually came to understand that our life at home without a father was different from that in a complete family. I even had the impression that they were less troublesome because of that. They didn't want to make it too hard for me. Eventually they even liked it that we were a threesome. Sometimes when they came home from a weekend at their father's they would say, "It's great that at home we have only one parent. At Papa's you always have to ask two people."

But they did enjoy the contact with Hans, who gave them lots of attention. They even went along with his family on holiday, and when they were older Hans sometimes took them abroad.

In those days we still had a large circle of friends, including some divorced parents with whom we celebrated Christmas and New Year's. That way the children didn't have the feeling that they were in an odd situation. Yet, sometimes Raf behaved strangely when he was quite young, although you could regard his strange behaviour at that time as a childish expression of something an adult has forgotten.

I remember that once after a rainstorm some kindergarten children cut worms in pieces with sticks on the street. Raf, who must have been about five, joined in. That night he dreamed about it. I was woken by terrified screaming from his room and got up frightened. Raf came to me crying. But even with his eyes open he couldn't rid himself of the dream.

"Wake up. You're with Mama," I said. But suddenly he ran away from me as though he were being chased and rushed through all the rooms of the house.

"Worms! Worms!" he screamed.

I picked him up and put him in my bed but he kept screaming. All the time he clutched my blanket with both hands and yelled, "Here too! There are worms here, too!" In every fold of the blanket he saw a worm. He kept jumping up, hiding his head in his hands and screaming the same thing.

"Now it's all over," I said after a while. "Now stop it." But it was as though he either didn't hear or see me or else he was asleep with his eyes wide open. Finally, once I shook him good and hard he became really awake, threw his arms around me and fell asleep again.

Around the same time he also had fits of rage if he couldn't get his own way. If we had to go home but he wanted to stay in the playground, he could have such a tantrum that I literally had to drag him along. At home he carried on with it. He kicked doors and walls, screamed and yelled. Then I took him in my arms and said to him, "Why are you acting so stupid? All the children go home when they have to eat." He snuggled against me then, still sobbing a bit. "Now try to be a big boy tomorrow and not cry when it's time to go home," I said.

After tantrums like that he would fall asleep exhausted. When he went to school and learned to read and write, which he did with great diligence, the tantrums stopped. But he remained an oversensitive child. When I read to him in the evening he reacted with fear at sad or scary stories and put his fingers in his ears.

Sabina worried about him. "Raf, here we go again," she used to say. "I'll let you know when you can listen again."

Raf took music lessons at a very young age: first flute, then guitar. He practised faithfully every day, preferably close to me and while I was drinking tea. It wasn't until he could be sure that I wouldn't go away that he began to play. I could see in his eyes that he was asking for compliments. It was soon clear that he needed me more than Sabina did.

He had a painfully excessive need to do everything as well as possible. He chose all his own clothes and if I tried to give him advice about it he would get angry. In that period it also struck me that he combed his hair for an excessively long time. Sometimes he combed it for an hour and was late for school. He got furious if I said anything about it and could not be dissuaded from his compulsive combing. He continually stroked his hair to check if it was still in place. In the end he would get anxious if anything came in contact with his hair. He would wear only sweaters and shirts that fastened with buttons. After a year this compulsion gradually lessened and finally disappeared. But his hair has always remained important to Raf. At the barber's he violently resisted having his hair cut, but because this happens a lot with little boys, I didn't pay much attention to it. Later I noticed that he distrusted people who made remarks about his hair. He has always continued to do that. He was one of the first to wear long hair and now it still comes down to his shoulders.

Although Raf and Sabina always played together, Raf still often took her toys. As the elder, Sabina was always the first to get a scooter, a bike, roller skates, or other important toys, and then it became apparent how jealous Raf could be. I promised him that he would get a bike the next year, but he couldn't bear to wait. On every possible occasion he grabbed Sabina's bike.

"I want to ride," he said and sped off.

When he was about nine he began to monopolize the shower so much in the morning that nobody else had a chance to use it. If we asked him to come out, he wouldn't answer and would lock the door. He emerged only when the supply of hot water in the boiler was used up. When I told him that the next day he couldn't be first in the shower, he answered that that was all right with him. He was somewhat ashamed, as though he himself was offended by his own behaviour. Eventually I succeeded in arranging fixed times for each of us. Raf couldn't resist doing something that he really wanted to do, and his compulsive fads kept coming out in other ways.

When I taught him French knitting he made dozens of yards of rope. He began very early while he was still in bed, and when I went to wake him I saw him feverishly knitting away. When that compulsive activity had disappeared a few months later, a new activity came along that he *had* to do over and over and that took precedence over everything else. He went fishing for hours day after day. When the season began he would become very nervous. The evening before he would lay out the rod, hooks, bait, and sandwiches and ask me, "Mum, will you wake me at five o'clock? You won't forget?" He was so enthusiastic that I had to promise.

He left at six in the morning, climbed into the shrubbery on the embankment behind our house and stayed there all day. He spoke to no one and only peered at his float; he would forget the time and I usually had to call him to come and eat. He kept this up for some years.

Once I asked him, "But Raf, how do you stand it – just sitting there all day long looking at that line to see if it moves?"

He thought for a moment, searching for an answer; he had a dreamy look in his eyes: "Oh, it's so quiet then, you can make up all sorts of stories. Sometimes it's as though they're quite real."

In the beginning of his time at the gymnasium a new interest came along. He began to read the books of Karl May one after the other and started acting like the heroes in them. He walked straight as a ramrod, looked at everyone with a penetrating gaze and did everything in a provocatively slow tempo.

At that time the difference between Raf, who was 13, and 15-year-old Sabina began to play a role. They gradually acquired differing interests and sought each other's company less and less.

Sabina became difficult and neglected her schoolwork. She went regularly to young people's cafés that were then springing up. But she couldn't handle all those new impressions. When I warned her that her schoolwork would suffer if she kept this up, she got angry.

When she finally failed a year, we decided that she should go to live with her father in The Hague for a while. Not only she but also Raf and I found that a difficult decision. In the beginning we found the house empty without her and it was hard to get used to her absence.

One evening I noticed that Raf looked tense and sad. He bowed his head as though trying to collect his thoughts. Then he began to talk thoughtfully: "You know, Mum, I've had such a heavy feeling recently. It's like there's something here." He pointed to his chest. "I often can't help thinking that I haven't been nice enough to you and then I feel guilty. Every day I'm dissatisfied with myself. It's one thing after another. At night I wake up and can't get back to sleep because I can't help thinking of things I've done wrong. When I get up in the morning I don't feel rested and at school I'm awfully sleepy."

Because I felt that he wanted to say more, I tried not to fill up the silence that ensued. After a while Raf continued, "There's something else." Again he paused. "It's hard to talk about it," he said slowly. "But I have to say it because it's worrying me."

There was another pause. I tried to encourage him. "Go ahead and say it," I said.

"My erections scare me," he went on. "My penis is too big and I'm afraid I'll never be able to go to bed with a girl. I can't help thinking about it a lot and it's causing things to get worse and worse at school."

"But Raf," I said, "You're imaging those things. Just read something about it and then you'll see that you're worrying unnecessarily. And as for your behaviour toward me, I think you're usually very nice to me. I remember that when you were about five, you said to me, 'It's a pity that I have such a dear little mummy. I'd really like to be a big, naughty boy but that's impossible.' So even then you were sweet to me."

I realized that I had neglected Raf for a while because Sabina had taken up so much of my time. He hadn't wanted to make it hard for me, but now that she was away I noticed how many problems he was struggling with that he had never talked about.

After this personal chat he shut himself completely off from me again. He passed to the third year class and then his depressive moods began to be more pronounced.

There were always friends around him who tried to cheer him up. They brought along their instruments and made music together. That helped, and when his illness became more clearly recognizable they still kept coming, until Raf wouldn't let them in any more.

Chapter 2   The Medical Education Bureau

The serious difficulties began when Raf was about fifteen. He was then in the third year at school.

I had to go to hospital for an operation and asked him if he wanted to stay with a friend of mine. He replied that he would rather stay at home because he was having a test and there would be too many distractions at the friend's house, but he would like to eat there in the evenings.

I thought it was a pity that he kept to himself so much. My friend's son was Raf's age and they were good friends.

When he came to visit me in the hospital a week later, he gave the impression of being preoccupied. He had also forgotten things that he was supposed to bring for me.

"Can't you manage by yourself?" I asked.

He looked dreamily outside and said shyly and apologetically, "I have a lot of homework."

When I came home I noticed that he was still more withdrawn than before. He spoke little and had a great deal of trouble with his homework.

When after about six weeks he came home with a girlfriend, I thought that she could be the reason for his strange behaviour. He introduced this girl to me and went with her to his room, where he stayed that evening.

From the time he was ten I had already noticed that he was greatly interested in girls. He wanted them to like him, but didn't want to try very hard to make them like him.

The following evening we sat together silently. Suddenly he began to talk: "I must tell you something else". He looked at me searchingly to be sure that I was paying attention. "When you were in hospital I went to a meeting of the Humanist League. I met a girl there who was slightly older than me, about 17, I think. The next Sunday she suddenly turned up on the doorstep without phoning first. I was pretty confused, because she immediately began to get familiar with me. After a little while she asked me if I would go to bed with her."

Raf had got contraceptives from his father, but as far as I could gather he had never yet had a chance to use them.

"I was nervous," Raf continued. "It didn't work. Then she began to laugh hysterically and said that she thought I was useless. I can't remember much more. It was as though everything was spinning around. There was a buzzing in my ears. When it was over I noticed that she'd disappeared."

He slumped in his chair and said wearily, "I don't want to do that any more. A girl shouldn't be so brazen and domineering."

After this conversation I became aware of how very tired he was. He spent hours on his homework, had more and more trouble getting out of bed in the morning, and literally fought with himself to pass to the fourth year, which he managed with great difficulty. But suddenly it was as though he had used up all his energy. For a week he stayed at home apathetically without doing anything.

One evening another girl whom I had seen once before came to visit him. When she left I noticed that something was worrying him again. He walked about the room nervously.

"Come and sit down, Raf," I said. "What's the matter now?"

"I don't understand why a woman wants sexual relations," he replied uneasily. "Surely there's no pleasure in it for her. It's humiliating when I long for something from a girl that doesn't do anything for her."

"Raf," I said, "you've got it all wrong." I asked him if he didn't know that a woman in this respect had about the same feelings as a man.

"Is that true?" he asked. "I didn't know that."

I got the impression that he was somewhat relieved.

"I'm glad you told me that," he said.

Later it turned out that this conversation hadn't helped. On the contrary, Raf went quickly downhill. He examined every problem from all angles, and he got into more and more difficulties with himself.

Hans thought he could still urge him on by promising him a motorscooter for his birthday. But after a while Raf also played truant from school and sometimes stayed in bed for whole days. At first he complained of stomach pain but later he stopped making excuses. The confidentiality with which he had told me about his difficulties had disappeared. Now if I asked him something, he pretended not to hear me.

In this way he muddled through that year, and for the first time he had to take the year over again. He had done literally nothing at school. His headmaster advised me to contact the Medical Education Bureau.

To my surprise they didn't take me into their confidence. The first time they spoke only with Raf. I felt abandoned. I didn't yet know what I should do. For the first time I got the vague feeling that I was being accused of something, but I didn't know of what.

Raf had a talk once a fortnight with a social worker who didn't begin a proper treatment for the first year. The people at the Medical Education Bureau probably hoped that Raf would grow out of his problems. And when he didn't get better, but rather became less and less approachable, he had a psychiatrist assigned to him and it was arranged that I should have a talk with the social worker every week. However, it seemed that I couldn't discuss the problems that I had every day at home with Raf. To some of my questions she gave no answer and she gazed at me without saying anything as though she wanted to hear from me what I wanted to know from *her*. She was secretive, as though she had something to hide, and I had a cool relationship with her. Nobody told me what they were afraid of. Still, I felt clearly that something serious must be the matter. The social worker was *so* careful, friendly and soothing that sometimes I was ashamed of myself. I wondered if she thought she was dealing with an under-aged person. I wanted to know how I should handle Raf when he said not a word, stayed in bed for days and received no one. But I was never once able to talk with her about my anxiety. It seemed that she held back and tried to distract me with things that weren't relevant. She probably didn't know how she could help me. She talked about a difficult crisis of puberty and said that I must have patience, and as a rule I went home with the same uneasiness as *before* the talk.

In the beginning I had some idea of the situation, but as time went on I thought that Raf didn't have much self-control, that he was too weak-willed.

"You must try to have a bit more spirit," I said. "If you fail this year again it's all over with the gymnasium."

He nodded and said wearily, "You're right."

But nothing changed. Finally I got angry when he didn't get out of bed. I could not bear it that he had changed so much in so short a time. At the same time I felt guilty, because I realized that he couldn't do much about it. I reacted with rage to drown my anxiety.

In the meantime Raf went more and more downhill. He rarely left his room. In the beginning of his decline he still took the trouble to get dressed and go to his psychiatrist, but after a while he stopped doing that, too. For days at a time I didn't see him, even though his room was adjacent to mine. He had locked his door and there was a lugubrious atmosphere in the house.

One evening I met Raf in the hallway. His head drooped on his chest. He walked very slowly as though he was dreaming.

"Can I help you, Raf?" I asked.

He didn't vary his pace. It seemed as though he neither heard nor saw me.

Since he no longer came to eat in the dining room, I saw to it that the refrigerator was full. At night I smelled fried eggs. If I went into the hallway I always saw a light burning and heard Raf moving around. He also kept his heavy curtains closed in the daytime.

After two months I phoned his psychiatrist and told him about the developments of the recent weeks.

"Can't you just come and visit Raf to see how he's living now while he's not coming to see you? Maybe you can help him?'"

"No, Mrs. Anstadt," he answered. "Raf must come to me himself."

"But you know that he doesn't come. He hardly knows that he's alive. You've been waiting now for months for him. Can't you just once come here for the hours that you reserve for him?"

I got a lengthy "Hmmmm..." for an answer. Then he said, "I'm sorry. That's impossible." With that our conversation was finished.

Raf left his room now only to get food or to go to the toilet. You could smell the stale air from his room in the hallway.

During this period, which lasted for about six months, he was out of the house only three times to get a breath of air, and then only at night. Then I would quickly go to tidy his room, open his window, and put clean sheets on the bed.

Of those three times, the police twice brought him home. In those days they were not so used to him yet, and Raf was conspicuous because he walked so slowly with his head down and didn't answer when he was spoken to. The second time a policeman came upstairs with us. He looked at me pityingly.

"How has this happened?" he asked.

I could offer no answer to that.

"Surely that boy must have help?" the policeman said seriously. But because I got no help, this remark only made me more miserable and hopeless.

During our conversation Raf stood in the room staring straight ahead and didn't react at all, as though it didn't concern him.

I lived with a ghost in the house who never spoke, but I persevered because I was still hoping for a sudden change. I understood less and less why the Medical Education Bureau had abandoned me. Both the psychiatrist and the social worker left me alone with a problem with which I was completely unfamiliar. Every direct question was met with a "Hmmmm" by the social worker. Quite soon she decided to suspend her talks with me and to resume them again only when Raf should visit his psychiatrist. And in all that time, she didn't once enquire about him.

ALL MY FRIENDS ARE CRAZY

A friend of Raf's who was determined to see him succeeded, after half an hour of knocking and talking, in penetrating as far as his room. During that visit Raf left his door open and I saw him silently lying on his bed with a pillow over his head. But no matter how calmly Raf's friend coaxed him, Raf could not be drawn out of his isolation. Later he often put a pillow over his head when he didn't want to be disturbed.

Another friend and classmate with whom Raf still had the most contact was received by him as though he were a total stranger.

"Raf, cut it out! I'm Frits!" he exclaimed.

But he got a chilly smile for an answer and went away terribly upset.

After a while I phoned the psychiatrist again to get him to visit Raf. Eventually, after I had repeatedly asked for help, he impatiently advised me to get in touch with the Area Health Authority if I couldn't cope with the situation. The tone in which he deigned to speak to me gave me the feeling that he thought I was being unnecessarily difficult, even though the hours that he had allocated for Raf up until then had been paid for in full by the Medical Education Bureau and by me.

The next day I phoned the Area Health Authority.

Raf must have heard that conversation, because when the psychiatrist from the Area Health Authority came and I went into Raf's room with him, he was dressed and had combed his hair and was waiting. I was speechless with surprise. He shook the psychiatrist's hand, and when he asked Raf how he was, he answered in a completely normal tone of voice, "Fine, Doctor. For a little while I didn't feel very good but now I'm OK again."

Then he asked if the doctor knew of a tennis club for him. "I want to take up sports again to get back into shape," he said.

After this short conversation the psychiatrist looked at me crossly and said that there was nothing wrong with Raf and went away.

When we were alone again Raf acted completely unconcerned. He said nothing; calmly pushed me out of his room, locked his door, and probably went back to bed. It was alarmingly quiet. I stood alone and pressed my knuckles against my temples. It had all happened so quickly. The loneliness and the helplessness in the face of so much lack of understanding gave me violent palpitations. Panic and a feeling of rage welled up in me.

After a good long cry I was a bit calmer. But I could not get rid of the memory of what had happened.

What kind of sickness was it where a person could change so? I wondered. How could such a friendly, calm, and intelligent boy that Raf had always been develop into such an emotionless, almost cruel, being so that he had become a stranger to me?

I realized that I knew nothing about his illness and also could not find the courage to discover more about it. I wanted to retain some hope, but yet the latest developments did not allow me to be calm and after some months I phoned the social worker again.

When I heard her voice, which always sounded so composed and friendly, I was angry.

"This is Mrs. Anstadt," I said in a formal tone. "I have waited long enough now. Why may I never talk to you and why don't you tell me what is the matter with Raf? You must have been through this before and know the symptoms. You are the social worker who was assigned to me. Shouldn't you be able to tell me what is in store for me? But you and the psychiatrist are completely abandoning me and haven't inquired once how Raf is."

"I understand that it's difficult for you," said the voice on the other end, "but at the moment we can do nothing for you. As the psychiatrist has already said, Raf must first come to talk himself."

I was baffled.

"But Mrs. Hendriks, it's exactly because Raf is sick that he doesn't go to his psychiatrist. He can't go in his confused state. Surely you know that!" I almost screamed.

"Try to be as calm as possible, Mrs. Anstadt. Perhaps soon it will get a little better. I wish you strength."

When she had hung up I realized that this conversation, too, just as that of the previous evening with the psychiatrist, had only the aim of keeping me out of everything. I got the feeling that everyone was conspiring against me.

The days at home were unreal. There was no sound. But in spite of my loneliness, I realized that I must still be happy that Sabina didn't live with me any more. There was no longer a place for her in these sick surroundings. At her father's things were going fairly well, although she had the same problems at school as here. When she came to Amsterdam she looked up her old acquaintances. She tried to make contact with Raf, but she couldn't understand the new situation and that frightened her. When she had gone away Raf had still been fairly well.

In the last weeks the atmosphere at home had become more and more oppressive. I felt more and more the need to talk to others about Raf's condition. Perhaps that would help me. Some of my friends found mentally ill people so creepy that they never even asked about Raf and were ashamed and irritated if I began to talk about him. But now I felt that I must nevertheless persevere so as not to become any more isolated, in spite of their aversion to this problem.

One day I suddenly heard Raf playing a Bob Dylan record that he often used to play. After that he took a shower, something that hadn't happened for weeks. The next day he came into the living room fully dressed and said that he was feeling better and in a few days would probably go back to school. I understood from that that he didn't realize how long he had lived outside reality and did not know that he hadn't been to school now for six months. He looked strange. He walked around proudly with his head up. His eyes, which had always been so wide-open; he kept almost closed.

"Do you have a headache?" I asked.

He answered in the negative but remained in this peculiar posture looking through the slits in his eyes.

I had already noticed that since his sickness had begun, there was nothing predictable in his behaviour any more. At times when he felt somewhat well he tried to do the things that had to be done and then suddenly he stayed in bed, sometimes for weeks, completely silent and without recognizing anyone.

After a week he suddenly came into the living room one afternoon with his jacket on and said, as though it were the most normal thing in the world, "I'm going to the psychiatrist's."

I then phoned the social worker, as arranged.

At my visit she now looked serious. "We have found it necessary to change Raf's treatment a bit," she said. "On reflection, the Bureau considers that it's not good to let Raf take part in group conversations as we had planned." But yet again nothing was explained to me.

This secretive behaviour on the part of the Medical Education Bureau social worker gradually made me feel that Raf's illness was of the kind that people preferred not to talk about. That gave me a feeling of inferiority that deprived me of the strength to be rebellious. When I had Raf at home again I wondered despairingly why people let me muddle along so without any help. An illness must surely be curable in a hospital or with medicines.

Raf had completely fallen back into his old pattern. He got dressed only late in the afternoon and now and then received friends. As time went on he again stayed in bed for days.

I read books about identity crisis, which the social worker had mentioned, and tried to keep my spirits up.

Chapter 3   Vacation

By now there was no longer any question of communication between Raf and me. He lived as if in his own world in his room, which he had decorated strangely. At the sides of his ceiling he had driven nails on which he had strung black woollen yarn from one wall to the other like a cobweb. The ceiling was thereby lowered by half a metre. On that yarn there were fastened at least thirty red tassels, which hung down so that Raf himself could barely walk under them without touching them. As the only sign of life I heard the same music over and over. Suddenly I understood why Raf looked so strangely through his half-closed eyelids. He held his head just like Bob Dylan on the cover of his last album.

Raf's friend Frits, who was received so coldly on his last visit, hadn't lost heart and one morning came to the door again.

"Is it you?" I said surprised. "I don't think Raf will let you in."

But this time Frits was not sent away. I even heard snatches of a conversation through the wall.

To my surprise Frits now came more and more often. There were even times when he didn't go to school and stayed whole nights, which Raf and he spent talking and playing records so loudly that I couldn't sleep. When it got to be too much for me I knocked and said, "Frits, you've got to go home now. I don't feel like these all-night parties. You can't keep on living here."

"I'm not visiting you, but Raf," he answered. "I don't have the impression that I'm bothering you."

He closed the door and I couldn't do anything else.

That same week his mother phoned and asked me to please send her under-age son home because otherwise she would have the police come and get him.

"Yes, that seems best to me," I answered, "because I can't manage it."

When the police came, Frits went with them quietly, but a few days later he was back with Raf again.

Summer came and Raf felt a bit less sick. "Frits and I are going to Sweden for this vacation," he informed me.

I was startled at first but when I had thought it over I was actually a bit relieved. I hoped that maybe a trip would do him good.

As the departure date approached Raf and Frits got more and more nervous. They would begin all over again to have doubts and get excited. The trip was postponed again and again. Raf constantly found new reasons to wait for another day. Their baggage grew until it could hardly be lifted.

The dithering got so irritating that one morning I said, "If you don't go now I'll throw your baggage out first and then you!"

Although I felt sorry for them, it seemed to me that now was the time for them to get on with it. They finally left.

The merciful rest after Raf's departure came to an end after a week when I had a phone call. "This is the police," someone said in German. "Are you the mother of Raf Keller?"

"Yes," I replied, alarmed.

"We came upon you son hitchhiking on the road and thought it wasn't responsible to let him go on. He seemed disoriented to us. Are you aware that he is out of the country?"

"Has something happened?"

They couldn't say.

"If you don't give permission for him to continue hitching, we'll send him back to Holland," they said.

I knew that Raf would not let himself be sent, so I answered, "Just let him go. He does what he wants anyway." After that I heard nothing more from or about Raf for the whole month. Only when he was back in Holland did he phone from Central Station.

"Can you come and get me, Mum?" he asked in a tired, flat voice. "I don't have any money left for a taxi and I can't walk because there's something wrong with my foot."

Relieved that I had heard his voice, I phoned a friend who had a car and we went to the station.

There stood the two boys. Raf's hand was in a sling and he was wearing only one shoe. He looked dishevelled and didn't seem happy to see me again. Nor did he say anything in the car. When we were at home he asked, "Could you help me? I want to put a plastic bag around my hand and my foot. I've hardly had a bath in all this time."

He seemed to be more confused and sadder than before he left. Also I noticed how blankly he looked at me. After a few days I still knew nothing about his trip.

"Say, can't you tell me anything?" I asked when I met him in the kitchen. "You broke your finger and burned your toe somewhere?"

"Oh, a trapdoor fell on my finger," he said unwillingly and peevishly.

"And your foot?" I pursued.

"A boiling coffeepot fell on it when I bumped into the cooker."

Another time he also let slip that he didn't like the director of the camping site.

Frits was no longer turning up. Again Raf slept during the day and walked around at night. One night, when I walked past the open door, I saw him sitting on his bed dressed. He was staring fixedly ahead and smiling with strangely shining eyes, as though he saw something beautiful in the distance. His lips moved. He was talking to himself, which I hadn't seen him do before.

Again he shut himself up and only went out once in two weeks to the hospital to have his finger treated. As usual, I took advantage of his absence to tidy up his room. When I opened the door a sinister, spooky atmosphere hit me. The first thing I noticed was the black cobweb ceiling with the red tassels on it again, but now the floor was also snowy with white threads carefully spread over the whole area. Raf's mattress, which had been yellow originally, was picked bare on the top side. A dark grey patch of foam rubber gaped open.

Raf must have been busy night after night, not only picking at his plaster bandage but also picking his mattress bare.

His doctor phoned to ask what on earth Raf had been doing with his plaster bandage. It hung in tatters around his hand and it had to be renewed every time. I told him something about Raf's illness and about the state in which I had found his room.

Communication between Raf and me had now become even more awkward. But once he did confide to me that after the vacation he would go back to school, which seemed unlikely to me, but I still wanted to believe it.

"Do they know that you're coming?" I asked. "It's been such a long time." He looked at me disdainfully.

"I'm going," he said in a measured tone.

The day before school began he collected his books together and carefully put them in his bag. The next morning he got up on time and had breakfast with me without saying anything. When it was time for him to leave, I noticed that he made no move to go.

"Raf," I said, "you must go now."

He looked at me again with that cold, almost devilish smile and said with gritted teeth: "Oh is that what you thought?"

Then I lost my temper.

"That does it!" I screamed. "I can't stand this horrible life any more! You've got to get over this and stop being so cruel!"

I stamped my foot because I still didn't want to give up the hope that I would be able to bring him to his senses. Up until then I had found an explanation for all his excessive behaviour.

I wanted to believe that he had dropped his guitar, which he loved to play, and not smashed it on the floor in a confused attack of rage. I wanted to believe that he couldn't get his door open and that was why he had had a bowel movement on a newspaper in his room. I could not handle it that in so short a time such a change had come over him. But now I wondered in my anger if I had really expected him to go to school. Because of the cold, defiant gaze with which he looked at me, I had no more room for pity. I felt myself become ice cold. An uncontrollable rage overcame me. I looked around, seized a heavy ashtray and threw it straight at his head. He hunched his shoulders and clutched the sore place with both hands without making any sound.

This movement suddenly had something human about it. A flash of pity went through me. I had an uncontrollable fit of crying and Raf suddenly acted again like the old ordinary, concerned Raf from before. He said in a friendly, sympathetic tone of voice, as if an old film were being run, "Mum, calm down." Then he said he would phone my brother.

Feelings of pity, guilt and exasperation were all mixed up inside me. I didn't know what to do with myself and couldn't stop crying, as if I suddenly had to get rid of everything. I took the telephone out of Raf's hand when he had called my brother and said, "You must come and get Raf at once. I can't stand it any more. I don't care what you do, but this has got to stop."

I could tell from his reaction that my brother had been expecting this. He came quickly. Raf was so frightened that he let himself be taken by the hand.

When my brother had taken stock of the situation, he phoned a friend who was in touch with a social work institution, and he made an appointment with her. I had the impression that they had already devised a plan in case things should go wrong at home.

Raf went quietly with Rudie, looked at me again for a moment, and said, "I hope you'll feel better soon, Mum."

After he left I started to cry again and could not calm down, especially because I felt so guilty about Raf, who had suddenly gone back to being so considerate.

My brother had phoned a friend who now came to see me, but she could not quieten me, either. She called my doctor.

"I'm giving you a sedative now," he said, "and when you are calm again I want to talk to you in some detail about Raf."

"All right," I said, but again I felt that I would rather be consoled than know the truth.

That same evening, my brother told me that I could put my mind to rest. "Raf is here in Amsterdam in a young people's boarding school where there was room for him. Now just see that you yourself catch your breath again a bit and as soon as you can, simply go to him."

When I visited Raf he seemed to have visibly improved in these new surroundings. He went to school again and was as helpful and friendly as before. Later it appeared that in every new environment he always recovered for a while, but as soon as he got used to it he fell back into his old pattern and created his world of hallucinations again.

He didn't talk about what had happened at home, as though he had forgotten everything. Only the plaster on his forehead was still a reminder of what had happened. But within two months he started telling the strangest stories about the boarding school.

"Mum, I have to get away from there," he said. "One of the boys is as strong as an ape. He keeps pestering me and always wants to fight with me. Yesterday he jumped up into the panelling of the ceiling and now it's hanging down, and that's not the half of it. I'm afraid that he'll smash my guitar. He keeps wanting to get his hands on it."

I phoned the school about it, but apparently that story was not true. In the end Raf could not stay because of his disruptive behaviour. But what I couldn't manage at home could be accomplished there. Now help came from the Area Health Authority, and they didn't let themselves be intimidated, as I had been. Within three months the authorities of the school asked my permission to admit Raf to a psychiatric institution. I agreed, even though this idea frightened me.

"It's becoming a difficult case," the director said when I phoned him to ask how Raf had reacted to his departure. "Raf is very frightened of going to the hospital, although we have prepared him for it. Because he's so uncommunicative we couldn't have guessed that he would be so afraid. When the Area Health Authority came this morning to pick him up, he locked himself in the toilet. We don't want to push him too far. So we've decided to postpone the admission. We shall see whether we can do any more for him."

The director was a gentle man and I trusted him. But I was perplexed by my own feelings. I had expected an eventual cure from this hospital admission, which was now postponed yet again.

I didn't have to remain in uncertainty for long. Raf now seemed even more difficult to handle than before, and the authorities of the school decided to go ahead with the hospital admission.

Chapter 4   Pavilion Three

Pavilion Three was the first institution where Raf was admitted. After a week we got permission to visit him, and I arranged to meet Hans and Sabina at the entrance. We rang the bell and in a little while we heard the rattling of a bunch of keys. Someone approached with quick steps and there was a moment of silence before we heard the door open.

On the inside the building looked old, dark, and gloomy. We had to go thirty metres down a hallway, and then it annoyed me that we had to wait there in front of a second door in the form of a gate for another ten minutes until it was opened for us. But in contrast to the first hallway, this one was very crowded. To our right we saw a large, dingy, dark room from which stale air drifted out to us. There were sixteen beds there. On the left-hand side were small rooms with one bed in each one. We could see through the open door that people were lying asleep in all these beds. Later we heard that these patients were undergoing a sleep cure.

Men and boys in white pyjamas like judo suits were walking in the hallway. A boy with a face covered in bruises who looked as though he had been in a fight spoke to us furiously. "Just look what they do to you here!" he said angrily. "They beat you up if you don't do what they say. Great little place."

"Surely that's not true?" I said, shocked. "They don't really do that here, do they? What happened?"

The boy looked at me fixedly and angrily and walked on without saying anything more. A moment later he spoke again, but only to himself.

On both sides of the hallway were placed benches on which men were sitting. Some were crying, others were laughing or swaying as if they wanted to rock themselves to sleep. A boy wearing make-up came past with angry little steps. He wore women's clothing and had a red wig on. His Adam's apple was conspicuously large.

"What's Raf doing here? He doesn't belong here," I thought.

At the end of this second hallway we saw rooms with small windows far above eye level that were blocked with bars. In one of those little rooms sat Raf. He received us furiously, pushed us outside and followed close behind.

"You've had your own son locked up in a madhouse," he said bitterly. "I'm not staying here. I want you to take me back with you."

The first impression that I had had of the institution gave me the feeling that he was right.

"It's just a short stay," said Hans with a voice that was constricted by nervousness. "You'll be home again soon." Sabina fought back her tears.

"Take me with you, goddammit, take me with you!" yelled Raf. "I don't want to stay here."

His voice cracked. I had hardly ever really heard him scream. He pounded with his fists against the unbreakable glass of a window in a door and began to throw around everything he could get hold of – chairs, ashtrays and vases – with the impatient rage of the loser.

His shouting changed into continuous screaming.

We stood there, not in a state to do anything.

Strong men in white coats appeared. They had a long folded piece of heavy, white cloth with them with which they bore down on Raf. The head nurse was also with them.

Raf tried his utmost to defend himself. "Go away! Go away!" he shouted and hit out in all directions. And then, "Mama, Mama!"

Finally there was just screaming. I ran away in panic, closed my eyes, stuck my fingers in my ears and squeezed into a corner as if I were trying to go right through the wall. My teeth chattered and I shook my head in order not to have to feel anything.

Raf's yelling faded into tired moaning. The head nurse came to me with a glass of water and a pill.

"Just take this," she said.

I saw that her hands were scratched open and bloody and I looked at her enquiringly.

"This happens," she said in an offhand tone of voice. "Your son has had to go through a lot in the last few hours. This outburst of rage was inevitable."

Raf still lay writhing on the floor of the hallway, fighting with the strong nurses. And now I just simply wanted to take him home and protect him. The sound of Raf's screaming and calling for help stayed in my ears for days and left me with a dull feeling of guilt.

On my next visit the head nurse asked to speak to me.

"I understand your anxiety about our harsh treatment the first day," she said with a calm voice that gave me confidence. "But that was necessary. During serious outbursts of rage there is a danger that the patient might injure himself, sometimes with more serious consequences than the measures that we must take to prevent it. Raf had an injection after you left and later slept peacefully."

I understood it. But then I went into Raf's ward again and saw him walking through the hallway like a caged animal. He seemed surprised that I, as a mother, had been able to betray him so. This understanding didn't help, and feelings of guilt and pity got the better of me once again.

I now went to see him daily. He was gradually behaving more calmly and expected to be home again soon.

The head nurse explained to me that he would first have to undergo a 14-day observation. During that time his behaviour would be monitored and discussed with the psychiatrist. There would also be a detailed examination.

"Raf is in what we call an 'examination' section,' the nurse explained. "Here little or no medicine is supplied unless it is absolutely necessary. By that means we try to get the clearest possible picture of the nature of the illness. This is also the reason that people get such a fright when they come in. The seriously disturbed people that you see in the hallway we can't help effectively in the beginning. Not until the psychiatrist has made a diagnosis can we proceed to an intensive treatment. That can happen temporarily in Pavilion Three itself, but also at home with medicines, or in a psychiatric institution outside the city where the patients can settle down. In that interval there can also be difficulties because the adjustment of the medication sometimes takes a long time. Not every medicine works in the way we expect."

About two weeks after Raf's admission I met the psychiatrist who was treating him.

"Raf is very reserved," he said. "I should like to have a talk soon with you and his father."

When I went to see him I told him in detail about Raf's childhood. I talked about Raf's need, even as a child, to withdraw in solitude and about my uneasiness that the absence of a father could have influenced Raf's later life. I had the feeling or expectation that by talking about it I could help the recovery along. "Actually, Raf was never a cheerful child," I said. "When I would go to tuck him in and make jokes with him, his happy laughter could be so touching that it was -- although I don't know why – painful."

"It is naturally difficult for a child to grow up without a father when he sees that other children have one," answered the psychiatrist. "But in the end there are a lot of divorced parents, and most children are not disturbed. Naturally, it was not favourable for Raf's development that the divorce took place. However, I suspect that we would have been presented with this illness whatever the circumstances. His behaviour, as you describe it, indicates that he has had problems since his early youth. Quite early on external impressions must have affected him deeply. He could not, as you say, bear sad adventure stories in books. In fairy tales there is a lot of cruelty. Most children can enjoy being frightened by it and as a rule suffer no ill-effects from it. On the contrary, they can use it to get their own aggression out of their systems. They learn quite early that what happens to the wolf in 'Little Red Riding Hood' belongs in another world.

"Raf has never been able to learn that. He empathizes too deeply with heroes and victims, and I suppose that he wasn't able to distinguish between fantasy and reality. As you said, he identified with the heroes in his children's books. He acted like Old Shatterhand and later like the pop singer Bob Dylan. That very often happens with children, but it seems to me that even then, with Raf that identification assumed serious proportions. The dividing line between I and not-I must have been only faintly delineated in him.

"It happens to everyone now and then that their fantasy world dominates them. Sometimes images from a dream stay visible for a moment after waking, even though we know that they cannot be. But for Raf when he was still very young the worlds of dream, fantasy, and reality were less clearly separated than with other children, as is also revealed in his dream as a five-year-old boy. Also later at school it seems that in spite of his intelligence his concentration got worse and worse. He must have been then – before you noticed it – already quite ill and so very occupied with the other world in himself that he could no longer comply with the demands that were placed upon him. Only through great self-discipline and enormous willpower did he manage to keep going for longer than anyone could have expected."

The psychiatrist's explanation made a great impression on me. All the same, I was still distressed that he hadn't let me keep the illusion that it was all less serious.

I visited Raf, who now behaved calmly again and had settled down, and it reassured me that he could summon up patience for the fact that the hospitalization lasted longer than he had expected.

But on one of my visits I noticed that he was in great confusion. "What's happened?" I asked. "Why are you so jittery?"

He tried to deny that anything was the matter, and with the greatest difficulty I just managed to find out what it was. All the tension had made him constipated; he had been given a laxative tablet, and in the morning was shocked to find that he had soiled his bed.

"I already feel terrible that I'm in here," he said, more to himself than to me, "and now this on top of everything else." He shook his head and looked sad.

Raf was going to be eighteen and wanted to celebrate his birthday at home. He had asked his psychiatrist's permission for it, but had not obtained it. A week before his birthday a nurse rang me up. I heard a business-like voice: "Will you please not come to visit Raf this week. He doesn't feel well and cannot have any visitors."

This sudden news shocked me. "But then what's wrong with him?" I asked.

"You can ask his psychiatrist about that, but he is not available at the moment. Just phone back in the morning."

The next day I again couldn't reach the psychiatrist. Now I phoned every day but was always brushed off. Finally I got a male nurse on the phone with whom I had spoken before, and he could understand my unease.

"The psychiatrist is off sick," he said. "He's the only one who gives information. I understand that you want to know how Raf is getting along, but I can't help you."

"But his birthday is on Sunday," I stressed. "We can at least visit him, can't we?"

"Just a minute and I'll ask if you can." After a short pause I again heard, "Just come on Sunday morning."

That Sunday we went with a bag full of presents to celebrate Raf's birthday. We had no inkling of the nature of Raf's illness and expected to find him in bed.

When we arrived in Pavilion Three the male nurse said seriously, "You can stay for only fifteen minutes. That's all Raf can cope with."

Even to this day I still find it incomprehensible that we were never informed about the reality of Raf's illness. When we went into his room I could barely suppress a scream.

Raf stammered a few indistinct words. His neck was crooked and his body was bent, which made his head sit at a wry angle. His fingers were spread apart and he could barely use them, as we noticed later. He looked like someone who was rigid in a convulsion. We noticed by his behaviour that he was aware of his condition. His eyes were dull and sad.

We wanted to unpack the presents to have something to do and to keep our shock under control a bit.

"No, no," said Raf. "I can't do it."

He came and sat by me, threw his arms around me, and asked, "Mum, what have they done to me?"

At the time I didn't yet know about side effects of overdoses of medication. In those days they thought that this could be beneficial. After our visit I wondered whether I had done the right thing by allowing Raf to be admitted. I felt uneasy about this treatment.

At home we didn't say much to each other. Hans quickly went back with Sabina to The Hague and I stayed by myself. I had a heavy feeling around my heart, and I had trouble breathing.

The next day the head nurse of the hospital phoned me. She said that Raf couldn't have any more visits for the whole week. "It's better for him. It's such a strain for him when you're there. That's too much for him at the moment."

After that week the psychiatrist, who wore a big white bandage over one eye, told me what had happened. "Because Raf had behaved in such a detached way, I wanted to see another Raf for a change. You know that I had not given him permission to celebrate his birthday at home. When he asked me if he could go away I saw my chance, and I said, 'You go home? Somebody who poops in his bed!'"

Raf had then flown at him in a furious rage and had given him a black eye. The psychiatrist had not expected this strength and aggression. Raf had had to be sedated with an injection.

"We had to keep him sedated for another week after that. Yesterday I visited him again and he was rather better. The first thing he asked was 'What happened to your eye?' When I told him, he could remember absolutely nothing about it. I have the feeling that all this has not been for nothing. The ice between Raf and me is broken. Now he probably has more trust in me because he thinks I'm a good sport for not being angry with him. That could be an opening for a more intensive treatment."

After my next visit I noticed that Raf had indeed recovered quickly. His eyes were open normally again, just as before. He walked with his head up and wanted to go back to school as soon as possible.

Still, I thought that he was being childish and clingy. "I want to live with Papa," he said on one of our visits. "I like the idea of being brought up by a man."

Hans reacted happily, but at the same time nervously, to this wish. "I think you've made a sensible decision, Raf," he said. But Raf's wish to live with Hans made a strange impression on me.

"Unlike his father, I don't think that things are really going well with Raf," I told the psychiatrist when I spoke to him briefly in private. "In all his openness I think that he is also acting strangely now."

"That's right, you're not imagining it," he answered and looked concerned. "Raf still needs a lengthy treatment. This sudden rush off to his father also strikes me as metaphorical behaviour. I want to talk to you and his father about it. If you have time, let's go to my room."

By now Hans had come up behind us. But because we didn't have the courage to find out the whole truth by asking too many questions, much remained unspoken. The psychiatrist probably understood that we couldn't yet handle the situation, and he put off for a bit longer what he had to say.

Raf would now be sent for a while to an institution outside the city with lots of fresh air and freedom of movement. Altogether, he was in Pavilion Three for four months.

Chapter 5 Schizophrenic

In the summer Raf was transferred to the new clinic near The Hague with lovely gardens and modern buildings. I visited him twice a week and was enthusiastic about the surroundings and his light, sunny room. But I had the impression that Raf himself longed to go back to Pavilion Three. He became quieter and again withdrew more and more into himself.

"Don't you like it here?" I asked anxiously. His answer surprised me.

"It's really great here. You can walk for hours, and yesterday we played football with a little group of people." It sounded as though he wanted to reassure me. Then he was quiet again as though he suddenly had to stop and think about something else.

On my next visit I noticed that he was going steadily downhill. After two months he was again clearly ill, but could behave rationally, thanks to the medication. He did not fall back as far as before.

I couldn't get over my disappointment easily. No one had prepared me for the fact that Raf might have a relapse. But I did suddenly remember the concerned face of the psychiatrist in Pavilion Three, and I understood that, at the time, out of fear of hearing an irrevocable verdict, I had denied him the chance to tell more about the course of Raf's illness.

The visiting hours now went by awkwardly. Sometimes Raf said nothing for a whole hour. I very often tried to talk to his new psychiatrist. I felt that in that way I could force a cure for Raf. I recall that I looked for a hopeful word in every nuance of his remarks. But he had nothing hopeful to report. He probably expected the worst but hoped, like me, for a sudden recovery. I had been told that this sometimes happened with this illness.

I heard the truth from my own G.P., whom I met at the home of some acquaintances. He asked me about Raf's condition, looked at me enquiringly, and perceived that I still hadn't been told the truth.

"Raf is schizophrenic," he said.

Because he saw that I didn't flinch but instead kept looking at him questioningly, he left it at that and didn't continue with the subject. Once again I didn't dare ask for details. When I told Hans, I finally understood from his reaction how serious the situation was. Horrified, he looked at me, opened his mouth as though he wanted to say something, then pursed his lips and staggered to the sofa to lie down.

Shortly afterwards I spoke with a neurologist friend about Raf. I heard the same thing from him. Raf was suffering from schizophrenia. He told me a lot about it. He probably wanted to prepare me for what was in store for me.

"The illness is called schizophrenia because that indicates that it's to do with a split personality," he said. "So far little is known about the cause. In general it is assumed that there is an abnormality in the brain and that hereditary factors play a part in it. Is there schizophrenia in your family?"

"Yes," I replied. "But it's rather distant family. A son of the brother of Hans' father became ill at the same age. He's now well into his forties. He never recovered and has spent all that time in a psychiatric institution."

My friend nodded. "Through great stress or overwhelming events, the illness, which has been dormant for years, can suddenly come to the surface. But very often the onset erupts without any reason. There are different kinds of schizophrenia. Sometimes the symptoms appear temporarily and it is possible that the patient can manage for a long time in the community. But Raf's illness, which is also called nucleus-schizophrenia, and which manifests itself around puberty, is the most serious and as a rule is incurable."

"I always feel so guilty," I said, "because I've had to bring him up by myself."

"You don't need to feel guilty. The illness would have come out anyway. It can be that Raf will sometimes feel well for long stretches at a time and will apparently lead a normal life. Then he will have more contact with the outside world, but at the same time he will keep his unreal world in himself and keep any appearance of it to a minimum. Over time he is going to hear voices more and more clearly and more and more often and will carry on conversations with the split-off personality in himself. You will notice that you'll be able to stop that in the beginning by distracting his attention."

He stopped and looked at me with great sympathy. "You must be prepared for this not to last," he continued. "His second ego, his split-off personality, will increasingly demand his attention and he will need his surroundings less and less. Often these patients become autistic in the end, turned completely inward. Sometimes this illness clears up around the age of fifty, but by then the patient has lost so much ground that he no longer fits in society, even though he's stopped having hallucinations."

After this enormous blow, which gave me violent heart palpitations, I gradually recovered, but I couldn't accept what I had been told. "Raf is not all that sick," I said to myself. "He'll get well, whatever I have to do."

Meanwhile, it seemed that Raf didn't feel at home in the bright, modern clinic. After a few weeks when he had said hardly a word, he began to talk again: "I don't like it that the nursing staff call me by my last name and use the formal pronoun '*u*' instead of the informal '*je*'," he said on one of my visits. I'm only just eighteen! Why don't they act normal and friendly?"

I had noticed how from the very first Raf had reacted uneasily to the formal treatment, but I thought that he would just get used to it. That complaint about addressing him with the formal Dutch pronoun was something new. It was meant to show respect for the mentally disturbed.

All in all, the surroundings were too low-key for Raf and the patients were too old. Fortunately, after a while someone his age came who also played the guitar and with whom he got along well.

His condition was changing all the time. Sometimes he behaved rationally when I came, but at other times he would be unreachable and living in his own world.

After a while he again stayed for weeks in his room and read nothing but the Bible. Then I noticed on my visits that he spoke to me as if he weren't my son but a stranger who wanted to be friendly to me. He used Biblical quotations in his speech and behaved in a markedly distant way.

He was left a good deal to his own devices and so he got ample opportunity to live in his hallucinatory world. At that time the psychiatrists were still proud that there was so much peace and quiet where before shouting and screaming could be heard from all sides.

"In the beginning, after World War II we had expected a lot from the new medications, which were originally meant for soldiers suffering from stress," Raf's psychiatrist told me. "When these medicines were administered to patients in institutions and had a surprisingly good effect everyone was delighted. They thought they were at the beginning of a new era in which they would be in a position to cure the mentally ill. We organized football competitions for patients who previously weren't in a state to do anything and now understood the rules of the game and could join in pretty well. Our work changed. The patient no longer needed to be locked up, but could now enjoy a certain degree of freedom. We no longer needed to be afraid that they would hurt themselves or others, because they were substantially less aggressive. Even better medicines were being sought and for a very long time they didn't give up hope of finding them. Alas, and in this I must disappoint you: up to now we haven't gone beyond rest, some relaxation and acceptable behaviour of the patients. All the medicines work only temporarily and have to be taken for the rest of their lives."

After a year the people in the clinic thought that Raf had to have contact with the community and had to try to spend his weekends at home. In the beginning that was difficult. We both tried too hard to please the other. Raf's possessions had gradually ended up in the clinic. He had nothing to do at home and behaved like a guest. The atmosphere remained tense. Once, when he came home again for a weekend, he kept his coat on and got ready to leave immediately.

"I'm going for a walk," he said.

"Already?" I asked, surprised. "Won't you drink something first?"

"No, I get nervous here. I have the feeling that you always expect me to tell you things. The first thing you always ask is how I am. You never start with yourself. The thing is, I don't have anything to tell about. Everything's just as usual."

After that he made a habit of going for long walks during the weekends, and on one of them he met a group of boys with whom he got to talking. At the table he told me about it. He looked happier than usual.

"They asked if I wanted to play in their band, here in the neighbourhood," he said. "In a youth club at the Concertgebouw. They're nice fellows, I think. One of them is in my class at school."

The boys took an interest in Raf and came to see him regularly when he was at home. Raf went with them to the youth club, where he felt comfortable. Now he looked forward to the weekends. As soon as he got home his friends were there. They didn't drop him when he got a bit worse and threatened to sink into apathy.

"I'm not going back to the clinic any more," he said one day.

"But you can't just suddenly up and do that," I replied. "In any case shouldn't you talk it over?"

I didn't manage to get him to contact the clinic. Considering that no clear improvement was to be expected there and also because after a long time Raf had friends again, it seemed to me a good idea that after a year and a half he should try to live at home again.

I had also recently heard stories from him that had made me anxious. Once he said that someone wanted to hang himself. "That guy asked me if he wouldn't be better to tie neckties together, because rope seemed to him so rough around his neck. I told him I'd never thought about it." I was struck by how calmly he said it.

His mind was made up. He refused to go back. Now I had to notify the clinic, otherwise they would miss him that evening and take disciplinary action. The psychiatrist was plainly annoyed, but Raf's stubbornness could not be budged. All his life he had done what he wanted and never let himself be talked out of anything.

I noticed that the friends who came to see Raf at the weekend were smoking pot. Raf had never smoked before that, but now I saw that he also took a drag when the cigarette came round to him.

"Since when do you smoke pot?" I asked when we were alone.

"Oh," he said, "I just take a drag because otherwise they'd ask tiresome questions."

But after a short while he let the cigarette go by as inconspicuously as possible. I think that smoking didn't taste good in combination with his medicines.

He now spent whole days with his friends, and for a year things went fairly well for him at home. He was now almost twenty.

Sabina also came to visit more often now because, as she said, Raf was somewhat more open. She was considering coming back to Amsterdam and moving into lodgings. She hadn't finished school, but she had been accepted by the Rietveld Academy and now wanted to continue with drawing.

One evening when Sabina and Raf were talking about pot, Raf said, "Drugs are completely unnecessary to get high. Before I went to the Delta Clinic, I just didn't sleep for a couple of nights and then I automatically got lovely visions. Once I saw everything in my room in wonderful colours, which gradually became a big fire in yellow, orange, red, and all kinds of blue and purple colours. Gradually those flames changed into figures. It was wonderful. Just like angels in the Bible. They flew slowly through the room."

"How can you stay awake for nights on end?" asked Sabina, amazed. "After going to bed late just one night I get terribly sleepy."

"I don't know. First you can't get to sleep and then you notice that you have lovely dreams as you're lying awake, and then you want to stay awake to see those lovely dreams again. Then you sleep for longer and longer during the day." He suddenly stopped and his smile disappeared. "Later on the dreams weren't always so nice," he continued. Again he was quiet and stared pensively straight ahead. Finally he said, "Now I'm afraid of them."

At that time I heard that one of Raf's best friends in the club had had an acute psychotic episode and had been admitted to a psychiatric hospital. Raf reacted to that with a serious depression. He almost stopped eating and again sat for hours silently staring into space.

After about two months a second friend also seemed to exhibit psychotic behaviour. In the beginning he, just like Raf at first, didn't get up in the morning and stayed in bed all day, even though for quite a while Raf kept waking him up in the morning. In the end only his friend was still awake at night, and because Raf had learned in the clinic to sleep at night, he now saw this friend only infrequently, too, and became lonely again.

Things turned out badly for this circle. Raf was probably attracted to the kind of people with whom he felt an affinity. He tried, for as long as possible, to keep in touch with the club and with the two friends who had now been admitted to an institution and often went to visit them.

The first friend recovered after two years and was discharged from the institution and tried to find strength with a group that was interested in Eastern philosophy. But the second got worse and worse. Raf kept in touch with him and tried to help him if he got the chance. It seemed that Raf himself was afraid of sinking with him into the depths. This friend never recovered. He still walks around the streets completely out of touch and talking to himself.

Raf now went quickly downhill. Problems kept coming up that he couldn't handle. He fell in love with a girl who was studying music. They went around together and also played music together, but she was obviously not in love with him. He often went to her and always came back in a bad mood and paced for hours around the room.

I was especially concerned that his medicines were running out. "You must go to the Area Health Authority," I said one morning when he was being restless again. "Ask if you can get medicines there because you don't have a psychiatrist any more who can prescribe them."

"I don't need any medicines," he replied.

I expected him to change his mind, because up until now he had taken his pills without any problems. But he did not alter his decision, and his behaviour was visibly getting worse. It seemed clear now that without medicines he could not stay at home. I tried myself to make an appointment with the Area Health Authority; I rang up and got the person in charge of the Mental Hygiene Department on the phone. She reacted so quickly that it seemed as though she personally knew the disturbed patients who had been admitted in her administration.

"Oh, does your little boy need medicines?" she asked sarcastically. "Well, he can collect them in the clinic you took him out of."

"But I *didn't* take him out of it. Raf won't go back," I said, shocked by the accusation. "He won't stand for it."

"When mothers have sons who won't stand for it, they have brought it on themselves. I have better things to do than to bring up your little boy. He can come in himself, and if he doesn't come he doesn't get any medicines."

"Raf is a minor," I said firmly. "He's becoming more and more difficult at home."

"You should have thought of that before, Mrs. Anstadt. Good-bye."

She hung up. The tears welled up in my eyes from so much lack of understanding from someone who surely must have known how difficult a patient like Raf could be. I didn't understand why she blamed me. From the beginning of Raf's illness I wondered why social workers, instead of helping me, let me down so.

After two weeks without pills, I couldn't stand the situation any more. Raf behaved more strangely now than I had ever seen him do. Before, he use to whisper to himself, but now when he hallucinated out loud he sometimes behaved aggressively too. I could decipher half sentences that he would first yell and then say almost to himself.

"That was actually…" I heard him say. After that came a few unintelligible words and then: "In the last world, where the sun doesn't damn well do it." He sat on the sofa with his head in his arms and I didn't know whether he was laughing or crying.

Again, he began to lie in bed for days, didn't speak, and reacted furiously if I asked him something. He took a shower four or five times a day. Sometimes he brightened up a bit towards the evening and would come downstairs to watch TV. Then he was often remarkably friendly, as though he weren't responsible for the other Raf, who at that moment was nothing to do with him. This made me hope again that he was better, but that same night he could walk again for hours in the hallway, play the guitar and sing loudly, as though there were no one around him who could be disturbed by it. I was sometimes afraid of that loud, unreal noise in the night. In these situations I wasn't able to get through to him. He looked through me as if I didn't exist.

I wanted to ring the Area Health Authority again, but I couldn't overcome my fear at the thought that I would get the woman psychiatrist from the last time on the line again. I kept putting off the call. But Raf's behaviour was getting more serious by the day. Also, the neighbours were now complaining about the racket he was making at night.

One morning I decided to phone anyway. I had to have help. Again I asked for the Mental Hygiene Department and was put through to a male psychiatrist who listened calmly to my story and made an appointment to visit me at home.

"Try to put up with it for a few more days," he said in a tone in which I clearly heard understanding. "When I see you we'll see what we can do."

"I feel helpless now that Raf doesn't use medicines any more," I said. "At first I still hoped that he'd recover, and I could draw strength from that." I began to cry. "Life is so hopeless now. I don't know where I'm supposed to get the energy to keep going. You are the first person who hasn't given me the feeling that I'm the one who has made Raf ill."

Although Raf had told me that he wanted nothing more to do with psychiatrists, Dr. van Aken did succeed in getting into conversation with him on the first visit. He asked Raf about his activities and didn't mention his difficulties. "Is it all right with you if I come again next week?" he asked.

Raf nodded and went to his room.

"For the time being I want to talk with you and Raf every week," Dr. van Aken said. "You can call me at any hour of the day if you find it necessary. Maybe together we'll manage to make things a bit less stressful."

The simple realization that I wouldn't be alone if I needed help gave me a feeling of security.

After a week Dr. van Aken came again at the appointed time, and in the conversation among the three of us Raf was less tense than I had seen him recently. When the doctor asked him about hallucinations, he said that he did have them but didn't go into details. I had the impression that he might have said more if I hadn't been there.

The psychiatrist even managed to persuade Raf to take his medicines.

After Raf had gone back to his room Dr. van Aken said, "We'll have to take it one step at a time. Eventually I'll get to know Raf better. But it will also demand a lot from you. I see that you're nervous, which I can well understand. At the moment I have no comfort at all for you, but I do advise you to talk with a psychiatrist yourself from time to time about your own problems. Perhaps after some time you'll be able to deal with the situation better. In any case, Raf needs understanding even though he gives little back. He is alone with his fears, and I hope to get him to the point where he can bring himself to talk to me about them.

"Hallucinations are often coupled with terrifying and sad, but also sometimes amusing, images. It must be difficult for Raf to keep all this to himself. Sometimes trees change into faces, with branches like fantastic horns. Pictures start moving. Sometimes figures climb out of them, or a hand comes out and tries to grab the patient. It's also possible that while he's talking to you, in his eyes you turn into an angel or a witch. But he won't be able to tell you what is happening inside him. I understand how difficult that must be for you, but all the same it's good that you know it. As a rule, facial and auditory hallucinations go together. So Raf sees not only strange images but is also spoken to by figures that wield great power over him. He's dealing with that now all on his own. That must be unbearable for him."

"But how does something like that develop, anyway?" I asked.

"In general, it is accepted that schizophrenia is an expression of a defect in the brain by which the consciousness of reality is disturbed. Our brains contain storage places for impressions. When we perceive or feel something, we can immediately give it a place. We have read, for example, that lightning is an electrical discharge. When we see lightning a connection quickly arises between what we experience and what we know. Our brain forms a complicated system that ensures that all impressions get their correct place in our consciousness. But also in what we call normal people those connections can be temporarily disturbed. So someone may be afraid in a certain situation (for instance going out into the street) while he knows that fear is unfounded. Then there's a short circuit between feeling and knowing. But with a neurotic disorder like that the correct judgement of reality lasts. With people who suffer from psychosis this connection stays disturbed, even though it can sometimes happen that they temporarily react normally. In a psychosis, feeling and thinking can no longer be separated. The inner and outer worlds overflow into each other. There are delusions and hallucinations. We can influence that process chemically by administering certain medicines. You've noticed, you told me, how well Raf responds to even a little medication. Unfortunately, we are still in the experimental stage with this."

When he was leaving we made a new appointment. It seemed that my doctor expected me to support Raf more than I had done up until then. But I felt that this would be too difficult for me and that before doing that I would quickly have to see about getting a psychiatrist for myself.

I made an appointment with the Institute for Medical Psychology. I talked about my domestic circumstances and explained why I needed help. "Could you wait for a while or do you think that you need a psychiatrist immediately?" asked the social worker.

"I don't know yet how a psychiatrist would be able to help me, but I do need help," I said in a tone of voice that even I thought sounded aggressive. It was as though I was blaming someone else for Raf's illness. The social worker looked at me attentively, wrote something down, and didn't say anything more.

Within a month I got word that I had to go see Dr. Heineman. During our first talk he said that I had got priority and asked some general questions to get to know me. At our second appointment I talked in detail about my family situation.

"You have few contacts outside the house, I gather," the doctor said. "It would be good if you would go out to work for part of the day."

"I also feel quite lonesome with only Raf for company," I answered. "My friends find it difficult to come over when he's here. Maybe I'll be able to bear the situation better if I'm forced by work to think about something else."

On the way home I already had a feeling of liberation. Very soon I managed to get a part-time job.

Now that I didn't see Raf for a few hours a day, I could get some distance on the situation and I got calmer. Raf became more approachable when he noticed that I no longer suffered so seriously from his behaviour.

"How's it going, Raf? Did you sleep well?" I asked one day as usual when I came home.

"Let's talk about you instead," he answered. "I think it's important that you're OK."

"Oh, I'm fine. I like my work. What do you mean?"

"I want to go in again," he said shyly. He held his head down as though he felt guilty.

"And are you afraid that I won't be OK if I'm alone?"

He nodded.

"But do you want to go in voluntarily now, just now when you're a bit better?" I asked, surprised. I'd never thought of this possibility.

He didn't take up my question.

"Mum, will you take care not to be alone too much?" he said.

The evening before we had seen a television documentary about Buiten Oord, a psychiatric establishment in Santpoort meant for young people from 15 to 21. The treatment there was based on the theories of Laing, which in that time were widely adopted. Laing was of the opinion that the source of the illness lay not in the patient but in society. The idea was to help young people through their identity crises in this institution.

I had the impression that Raf wanted to have himself admitted in order to find a solution for his loneliness. On the following visit from his psychiatrist Raf said that he wasn't making any progress in this way. It was his aim to finish school eventually and go to the conservatory. That conversation made me realise that he had no idea about time. He was still always talking about his school as if he hadn't left it five years ago.

"I just want to have some friends again, too," he said. "I'm at home now the whole day. Alone. Now my mother often isn't there, either."

"That seems a good idea to me," answered the psychiatrist. "I'll submit an application for you as quickly as possible."

Raf soon got word and within two months he had to go for a talk in Buiten Oord. If the management and the patients had no objection, the admission could go ahead. I wasn't afraid of a rejection because Raf always behaved calmly and with great assurance. Even though he didn't go out of his way to make a good impression, people still liked him.

On the appointed day he went to Buiten Oord to introduce himself. When he came home that noon he said nothing, but he looked almost cheerful. It was only during the meal that he began to talk about his visit.

"It's nice in Santpoort, just like being on holiday. They play guitar, listen to records, and go on long walks together. They're all people my age. The Buiten Oord place hasn't existed for very long, they say."

"Do you think that you'll manage to go there?" I asked.

"Oh yes, those people are great."

Every time when he behaved so normally I would be buoyed up by the hope that he would get better. Maybe he would get better in Buiten Oord with people with similar problems.

Chapter 6 Buiten Oord

Raf was admitted in the spring. When I went to visit him after a fortnight, he looked radiant and said that he intended to take up his schoolwork again. "A lot of people here just go to school in Santpoort. I want to do that, too."

He swam a lot, he said, and they often played football – even the girls. They regularly took walks all together in a group to the beach, a walk of more than two hours. "I'm staying here until I feel completely better," he said contentedly. I looked at him. I was glad that things were going well for him, but it already pained me that his happiness could disappear again.

He was in a good mood for months at a time.

"Mum, come upstairs to the creative therapy," he said on one of my visits. "You've got to see what I'm doing. The therapy leader is there now, so you can meet him, too."

The therapy loft ran down the whole length of the building. There were unfinished projects sitting around everywhere. Many of them looked somewhat sinister. Among them there were drawings that at first glance seemed incomprehensible but that frightened me when I had a good look at them, for they expressed so much overt aggression.

At a table stood a thin man with a friendly face. I introduced myself and we chatted a bit. Then he took me on a guided tour. He said nothing about the content of the work.

"They are enjoyably occupied here," he said. "The people can indulge their emotions if they need to. Sometimes that does them good. In the afternoon there is officially no therapy, but Raf has recently been coming by himself to work anyway." He turned to Raf: "You're really keen, aren't you?" he said.

Suddenly I was standing in front of a big wooden bird, about a metre high, with a head made out of several different blocks. The feet weren't finished yet, but they were skilfully sketched out.

"That's what I'm working on," Raf said. He gave me a questioning look, as he used to when he was studying music and expected compliments.

"How marvellous, Raf," I said, and I meant it. "What an enormous job that must be to gouge that out of one block."

"The seven sensory organs are in the head," he explained. "The three holes that I made are painful. Those upper two are the eyes that he sees too much with, and the third is the heart. That is heavy and sad."

I looked at the therapy leader to see how he reacted, but he didn't say anything. Raf showed me more drawings. I found them impressive. They were done in black, deep red and orange. They all had the same dark horizon, with heavy rainbows.

Did Raf then not feel as well as he looked, I wondered? His work and his remarks about it had shocked me. They made me see clearly that he was letting his bird express what was going on in his mind.

For the first time in months I went home in a melancholy mood. I knew that I had once again deluded myself with something I wanted to believe. Raf remained fairly well adjusted for a while. I got the impression that he wanted to keep his problems hidden for as long as possible. I hoped that he wouldn't notice that I was again uneasy about him.

A couple of weeks later we were walking along the extensive lanes of the institution. "Raf, what's happening with that school where you wanted to go?" I asked. "Have you done anything about it yet?"

"Oh, no. It's so busy here. You can't concentrate on schoolwork. There are so many therapies. It begins in the morning with meetings of patients and staff. All the patients and the staff members sit in a big circle in the ward. Everyone can bring up new ideas and say what's bothering him or what he would like to have changed. That lasts from 9:30 until 11:00. After that, one group goes to do drama. They call that 'psychodrama'. They act out their own problems and some boys or girls start crying. I don't feel like crying. I don't take part in sad things. Then you still have to talk to the social worker or the psychiatrist. But it's so big here. If you don't want them to, nobody can find you."

In fact the building was too big for the 60

people who lived there. There were rooms and wards that were standing empty. The first time I was there it had struck me how beautifully cared for everything looked; modern, with bright colours. In the huge hallways stood big leather sofas. The lay-out made it seem that it had been originally established for more people. I had asked the management about that, and they had told me that it had been the plan to put 90 people in Buiten Oord but that they couldn't get the staff.

All summer I visited Raf every week. Sabina sometimes came along. In the meantime she had found a room in Amsterdam. She was happy that she could talk to Raf again and refused to accept the seriousness of his illness. "I know lots more people who've been in a clinic and now have got better again," she said.

I could understand that. I knew how long it had taken me to come to terms with everything. And even now I sometimes still had hope.

"Why don't you come to Amsterdam sometimes?" I asked Raf. "They'll let you leave, won't they?"

"Oh, I have everything here that I need," he said. "My friends, too."

It was just as well, I thought. In Amsterdam he could be influenced by other friends and perhaps, as had happened before, wouldn't want to go back to the clinic.

Around the end of the autumn when Raf had already been in Buiten Oord for nearly a year, he began to get quieter. He didn't look so bright now as he had in the previous months and was yet again withdrawn in my presence. It was harder and harder for me to get him to talk, and the visits became more uphill work every week.

I talked about it with the staff. They didn't find it alarming.

"At the moment Raf is going through a difficult period," they said. "He takes part in the therapies less and less and we have noticed that he roams about in the dunes for hours on end."

"But what do you do about it?" I asked.

"Up until now he has kept coming back. He will have to learn to ask for help if he needs us."

I felt powerless. In Buiten Oord medicines were given only in exceptional cases. But because a lot of work was done with patients as a group, as soon as he felt a bit better Raf was drawn into the group. Perhaps that's why his first relapse in Buiten Oord didn't last so long. But after that his moods kept changing. Sometimes he was lucid and took part in activities, and at other times he would be confused and quiet.

On one of my visits I couldn't find him anywhere. No one knew where he was. I looked in the big building and finally found him in the corridor, where he was sitting on the floor next to a seat. He didn't recognise me and was talking out loud in indistinct, incoherent sentences.

For a year he had managed all right. He had been one of the first patients in the original group with which they had first worked with much energy and faith in the new therapy. But now I noticed that it was going badly not just with Raf; the whole surroundings exuded a different atmosphere. The accommodation that was originally so cheerful had become somewhat dingy. Most of the residents were no longer so enterprising as they had been the previous year. I noticed on my weekly visits that the management, which consisted mainly of young people, did everything to discover where the difficulties lay. Although in their view society and the parents had made their children ill, they now wanted to organize consultations with those same parents, together with the patients.

Most of the parents came to the appointed meeting. Many of them looked anxious, helpless and confused. They knew little about the illness of their children, who in the meantime in Buiten Oord had adopted the language of the social workers.

It was made clear to them how they should behave toward their parents. And without holding anything back, one accusation after another issued from the microphone. Some children really didn't even want to be present on this "aggravating" family afternoon.

The parents scarcely had a chance to say anything. Only a few children went to sit with them. I had the impression that some would have liked to, but kept a stiff upper lip in front of their fellow patients. I took part in three of these pointless gatherings. Often the parents left the group event with tears in their eyes.

The patients now stayed away from creative therapy. Only required therapies could still be continued, but fewer and fewer patients came to them, too. The staff looked very diligently for the cause of the difficulties and still hoped to escape a crisis.

Raf didn't take part in anything any more. They let him alone, and I wondered what the point of that was. At first I thought that they had kept him in Buiten Oord for so long in the conviction that he could be helped. But as he cut himself off, he was left to his own fate. He was hallucinating now more and more. He even found it enjoyable. He liked the big corridors where he could walk around for hours without bothering anyone or being bothered.

After a year and a half a situation had developed in which nothing more was expected of him. He just went along with them and when he felt well he played the guitar in a little band that was formed.

But the difficulties in Buiten Oord didn't end. On the contrary, they got worse and worse. Increasingly it seemed that many patients, like Raf, could not be helped. I was surprised on each subsequent visit at the extraordinary state of things there. One time there were dozens of cups that had been smashed. Everyone stepped calmly over them.

"What's happened here?" I asked, surprised.

Raf just shrugged and said, "Somebody got angry."

"As angry as all that?"

He smiled. I think that he found my reaction touching.

"But why does everyone just leave it lying around?"

"Because it's nobody's concern. It's the business of the one who did it."

I probably asked too many questions and he found this too tiresome, because all at once he went away and didn't come back.

On my next visit there were windowpanes that had been smashed, and curtains and wall decorations hung in tatters. It looked sinister, especially because nobody was surprised at anything. It was as though that was the way it was supposed to be. I also sometimes saw trails of blood on the floor. Raf told me that more and more patients tried to commit suicide.

"They look for glass and cut their wrists, and when it starts bleeding badly they get scared and run to the group leaders." He said that with a gentle, resigned look.

Now that I was more attuned to it, I did indeed see boys and girls with bandaged wrists. Later it appeared that there were also a few successful suicide attempts. Many young people must have felt very abandoned here in this big building. Only for a few like Raf was this space an advantage. Here he could relax. No one paid attention to him when he walked back and forth or talked to himself out loud, just when this home was now having so many problems. Once when I had to go for an appointment, the ten doors of the consulting rooms were bashed in. There were holes in them that were bigger than a dinner plate. In the spacious, light corridor, where it was as quiet as if the section were uninhabited, these broken doors looked depressing. I wondered how anyone could get the chance to destroy so much. It must have been done with an axe.

I spoke regularly with my psychiatrist about what had been happening lately in Buiten Oord. "Whatever has suddenly started going on there?" I asked. "It's going from bad to worse."

"That doesn't surprise me," he said. "The Buiten Oord team is working according to the theories of Laing, an English psychiatrist who has a great following at the moment. He not only blames the parents and society for making young people mentally ill, but he thinks that they have to be accepted in their otherness. They must be admitted into the community. Laing also rejects the use of medicines. Buiten Oord wants to serve as a model for this theory. With that aim, the management has taken an impossible task upon itself. The disturbed patients are extra sensitive to atmosphere. If someone has a psychotic episode and goes and smashes everything up or makes a suicide attempt, the situation escalates and other patients are affected, too. That's how the situations that you encounter there have come about. They won't get that stopped without medicine."

"But what do you think is going to happen

there?"

"I'm sure that Laing's theories won't hold up. He has in a certain sense done good work by demanding a more humane treatment for patients in clinics. But I question the honesty of his motives. All I can say now is just that the theory of accepting disturbed behaviour is easier than trying to do something about it. But it's still too early to make conclusive pronouncements about it. Psychiatry is in a developmental phase. I'd be glad if you kept me posted about the course of events in Buiten Oord."

Under the influence of the internal troubles, more and more frequent conferences were conducted with the parents, which as a rule passed off especially discouragingly and resembled a diversionary manoeuvre. I was also summoned by the psychiatrist.

"Raf's getting along well, isn't he? Why is he here and not at home?" he asked me.

"But he asked to be admitted himself," I said, surprised. "And nothing has been said until now about discharge."

"Because you haven't put in a request for it."

"No, because I don't know what your reasons are for saying that Raf is getting along well. Either you are badly informed or you don't want to know that Raf has regular relapses. He has felt a little better now for a fortnight, but you know as well as I do that this can change in a few days."

"You wouldn't mind that, would you, Mrs. Anstadt?" said the psychiatrist now in an aggressive tone of voice. "Better your son cowering in the clinic than with you at home. Here you find him nicely put away, I notice."

"Doctor, you haven't seen Raf in his sick state at home. He sat all day sorrowful and alone. He gradually lost all his friends because he never left the house. And he likes it here and has people around him."

"Then you must let him live alone. Then he'll have to go out, otherwise he'll have nothing to eat. But you won't do that, will you?"

"If you think he ought to live alone, then it's up to him to talk to you about his discharge. Or do you think that I, as his mother, have to sort this matter out?"

Why did he attack me so? I wondered. After all, in the six years of his illness Raf had spent three and a half years at home. And apart from that, hadn't he himself wanted to be admitted? I couldn't help thinking of the conversations with my own psychiatrist and the theories of Laing, who always laid the source of a disturbed mind at the parents' door.

"But Doctor," I said angrily, "you don't know me and yet you make a snap judgement about my behaviour towards Raf. I'm seeing you for the first time. I find it offensive that I keep getting a different psychiatrist to talk to, who is instantly ready with accusations. What do you really know about the difficulties at home? Whole families are destroyed because they have to live with someone in their midst whom it's impossible to live with. You want to send Raf to Amsterdam and have him live by himself, which naturally won't work. That's why there are more and more families under strain, and so people have to be admitted to hospital again."

"That's not the way it is," he answered pedantically. "It is the family that destroys the mentally weak family member."

A conversation like that made me despair, because I didn't feel in any state to explain to others how a patient like Raf behaved at home. When Buiten Oord, with so many employees, wasn't able to restrain people from destructiveness, aggression and suicide attempts, how was a family supposed to do it?

Because of the internal crisis, they began to try out a reorganization with a new timetable. Patients whom they considered suitable for it were sent on a long week-end leave to prevent their being hospitalized in Buiten Oord.

Raf was now sometimes pressured by the staff to go home. He would always bring the same friend with him, a student who was not incurably ill and after a time recovered and went back to university. He still often came to visit us.

After Raf had been home a few times he stayed away again without being in touch at all. When I phoned him he said that he needed to be alone. I asked the authorities what the matter was. I was told that Raf had suddenly started behaving so inexplicably, going off whenever he wanted and sometimes staying away for days without telling them, that they didn't yet know what to make of it.

"But then don't you go to where he might be?" I asked anxiously.

"We can't go looking for him all over The Netherlands."

"But when somebody runs away, don't you look for them at all?"

"No, Raf is here on a voluntary basis."

But even though by now he had taken to staying away for weeks, he could still go back to Buiten Oord. More and more often now this urge to roam overcame him. No one could stop him. As a rule he came back hazy, I was told. He could remember nothing about the time he had spent roaming.

But however he felt, through it all he remained dedicated to his music and was regularly occupied with writing songs and playing the guitar. In his hallucinatory mode these songs had a fairy-tale, cryptic content. He wrote about love, the sun, about the past and future world, and about beings that occupied a kindly place in it and foretold a comforting future. In his imagination he was still the leader of a band and he talked about it as though it had been performing in the country for years.

In those days he had a great devotion to a certain female pop singer. At home he had often said that he wanted to visit her because he had written songs for her. One day when he had suddenly disappeared from Buiten Oord again, it turned out that he had gone to her. Because she wasn't at home and he wanted to present the songs to her in person, he waited the whole night on her doorstep. When he came back again the next two nights, the neighbours began to feel sorry for him and let him sleep at their house. They asked him where he came from.

"I live in The Hague with my father," he had said. "I'm studying music. It's important to me that Minda gets the music that I've written for her."

The neighbours phoned Hans. He came at once and asked where Raf wanted to go. "To Buiten Oord – that's where I live, isn't it?" he answered. That was all he said.

His behaviour now got to be the way it was in his most difficult time at home. There were periods when he did absolutely nothing, stared glassily straight ahead, and stayed in bed for days, sometimes weeks. During the visiting hours he often looked at his watch and then said that I had to leave. At such moments he couldn't control his hallucinations. He didn't want me to notice that and kept going off to one side to say something to himself which I couldn't make out. I did hear a few swear words like "damn it" and "not happen if..." He then looked furious when he returned. This self-control probably took a huge effort.

It didn't seem right to me that in this condition he was treated in the same way as patients with a completely different set of symptoms.

With the weekend approaching, the

institution authorities phoned me and told me that for the time being Raf didn't want to have any more visits. I resigned myself to it for two months and again hoped for a gradual recovery. But at the end of that time when the nursing staff still couldn't give me any information at all, I became increasingly concerned.

My psychiatrist advised me to let things take their course for a bit longer. "Anyway, you can't get through to him when he's in this state," he said.

Driven by anxiety I finally went, without Raf's permission, to Buiten Oord. By then I had not seen him for three months. With difficulty I was let in to see him. When I opened his door the foul smell took my breath away. Spider webs hung all over his room. The floor was strewn with fruit peels, ashes, cigarette ends, and partly eaten sandwiches. Fat flies buzzed around, and groups of them had settled in various places. Raf's sheets were almost black from the filth, and dust lay in a thick layer over everything.

I saw that in all that time no one from the nursing staff had been in his room. I saw that Raf was seriously ill. He looked at me with a vague smile, as though he felt at home in these surroundings. When I just put out my hand to make room for some candles that I had brought with me, he said in a dreamy tone of voice, "You mustn't touch anything here. Everything must stay the way it is."

"Do the nurses think that, too?" I asked to get a bit more out of him.

But he repeated, more to himself than to me: "Everything must stay the way it is."

After I had been with him for about an hour in the room where I was barely allowed to sit on a chair because this rubbish probably represented a magic power for Raf, I went to the group leader.

"Raf will get sicker and sicker in this room if nothing is done about it," I said.

"Raf himself is responsible for his room and he must clean it up himself," she answered.

"But have you actually been in his room? It's an utter pigsty in there. That surely can't be healthy? You do know that in his serious condition Raf isn't bothered by it? But his delusional behaviour will only get worse because of it. This filth will make him sicker and sicker. I wasn't allowed to touch anything in there. He lives as though in a sacred palace of garbage. He has got to have help!"

The group leader looked at me superciliously, but she said nothing more.

"Really, if you help him he'll perk up a bit again," I said, still with some hope.

But she still didn't react.

For a long time nothing changed in this situation.

It had now become clear to me that Raf was indeed going to have to go through everything that Laing had described in his books as a form of healing. Because I was getting more and more anxious, I wrote a letter to his psychiatrist and I asked *him* not to abandon Raf to his fate. I received no answer. My own psychiatrist was getting anxious about me, but he knew that he couldn't help me. He didn't dare tell me everything that would still have to happen to Raf before he could count on help.

I phoned the clinic every day. That's how it became increasingly clear to me how inhumanely social workers could behave because they believed in a new theory. "Mrs. Anstadt," I was told over the phone, "Raf still gets out of bed to eat, so we needn't give up hope yet."

But after a while Raf didn't come to eat anymore. The authorities stuck to their guns. They thought they could use hunger to force him to come downstairs. But when they noticed that this theory didn't work for Raf and he didn't appear, they finally felt that something had to be done. I don't know how long he lay in his room without eating. I asked my psychiatrist what he thought should happen.

"That is a sad way to treat people," he said. "But it's all according to Laing's theory."

"But what are they going to do with him?"

"Laing thinks it's good if the patient regresses totally and so becomes child-like. According to his theory, the cause of all mental difficulties must be sought in the first years of life. Patients often go so far back to their childish state that they behave entirely like a baby. They put their thumbs in their mouths, babble like a small child, soil themselves, and in the end don't know that they have to eat to stay alive. It is not known whether these patients have moments of lucidity when they realize what state they're in. That's also why I think it's wrong to abandon them to their fate. The anxiety that it provokes may cause even more damage than whatever happened in their youth. You cannot help Raf any more now that he has reached this stage. They will have to look for a solution pretty fast now in Buiten Oord.

"Alternative psychiatrists are of the opinion that a cure is possible without medicines. The reason for Raf's situation is that he didn't get medication in time. According to Laing, Raf must get over this serious regression by himself. Laing thinks that this experience effects a healing. It has recently become known that he has placed disturbed people, often children of rich parents who could pay for the expensive treatment, in ordinary residences, so that the parents don't have to suffer the disgrace of their children being in psychiatric institutions. Those disturbed children were seriously neglected there without any supervision. Psychiatrists rarely went to visit them. When they did go, sometimes the patients had already got into such a serious condition that their psychiatrists were no longer allowed in. In some residences patients lay soiled in their beds and were no longer in a condition to ask for help."[*]

---

[*] This situation was described in a series of articles by Johanneke van Sloten in the *Haagse Post* beginning in September 1980, entitled: "The Reality of the Anti-psychiatry in Ronald Laing's houses".

One day, when I again enquired anxiously how Raf was, I got a group leader on the phone that I didn't know. He said that he had only worked in Buiten Oord for a short time. His voice sounded friendly. "Yes, Raf has been very ill. I don't know him very well yet, but I've helped him to clean up his room. After all, we had to start somewhere. Raf felt a bit better after that. We'll help him get back on track."

I immediately made an appointment with this group leader to visit Raf.

"I believe that they've let me lie here for a long time without eating," Raf said when I was with him. By now I hadn't seen him for six weeks. "Nobody ever came to see me. I remember that in the end I just pooped in my bed. I've forgotten exactly how all that was. I recall too that in a corner of my room there was a pile of stinking sheets. They weren't taken away."

He looked pale, was very thin, and stared silently into space with a surprised smile. After a while he said, "Why do people treat each other like that, anyway?"

I wanted to pamper him, to make up for what had been done to him and to make him feel less lonely. Abruptly I asked, "Would you like to go home again, Raf?"

"No," he said. "I want to stay in Buiten Oord, although I don't understand why they did that. But now they're all really nice to me."

I understood that their method stemmed from their vision of Raf's illness. The group leaders still denied that it could be of a permanent character.

Sabina sometimes came over to ask how Raf was. She had a much more rebellious character than he and could not understand why he still wanted to stay in a place where they had treated him like that. She was in constant inner conflict about Raf. On the one hand, she was concerned about him and wanted to know about his situation, but at the same time she resisted too much information. Sometimes when she was eating at my house and I started talking about Raf, she would say, "Let's talk about something else for a change."

During this period in Buiten Oord Raf became increasingly difficult. He did what he wanted and was confused and angry. Sometimes he came home and stayed for as long as it suited him. Nobody from Buiten Oord called to ask about him. Once when he was in Amsterdam again, he was going around with impossible plans and bringing all sorts of strange people home with him. I was at my wit's end and phoned Buiten Oord to ask what I should do.

"If you let Raf in, that's your own responsibility. Then you are interfering with the treatment. But like all mothers, you want to have your son back and shift the blame for his behaviour onto the institution. If you don't let him into your house, he'll be obliged to return to Buiten Oord."

But could I do that? I wondered.

It was now summer and fine weather and I was working at home. For some reason that I still don't understand, I looked outside. I saw Raf coming shuffling along and I felt my heart start pounding. I saw from his foot-dragging that he was in a bad way.

Now stick to it, I thought.

The doorbell rang. I remained standing stock-still. The bell went again. I stayed motionless behind the curtain.

Raf walked to the little square. His head rose slowly, toward the window behind which I stood, and then lowered again. His body slumped. He started to go away but turned round again and looked up once more. I saw his shoulders rise in a deep sigh. Finally he went away. I stood there behind that window for a long time as though paralysed.

Chapter 7   Mrs. Raas

After a stay of two and a half years in Buiten Oord, Raf had to be literally evicted. He got to be too old for this institution, and gradually he could no longer be maintained without medicines. That he became increasingly ill didn't fit into the view the authorities had that schizophrenia didn't exist.

Raf was furious that he had to leave. He lived one day at a time and had never realized that he would have to get along without these surroundings that he found so safe. But when I compared him with other patients, who after a stay of a year and a half to two years got a panicky feeling of anxiety and abandonment when they had to leave, I found Raf's reaction not really so bad.

Some of them seemed no longer in a condition to get along in society after they had lived protected and almost without restrictions in Buiten Oord – an unreal world where anarchy reigned. Most were completely dismayed when they were told to get ready to leave. They needed the trusted environment of their fellow patients.

They were not the ones who claimed that mentally disturbed people had to have their freedom. They knew the nighttime fears of being alone with the hallucinations that were sometimes unbearable. They were told that independence was good for them by the hospital authorities, by the welfare workers – by the healthy.

A great many of these young people were

ordered to learn to live alone in rented rooms. The parents were advised not to take their children into the house, so that they could work together on a process of letting go.

People whom I knew from the clinic I later saw walking around in the city, lonely, increasingly neglected, with anxious, questioning eyes. Others shut themselves off from everyone else, in no state to stand up for themselves. One of the patients went to live on a boat after being discharged from Buiten Oord. It was also impressed upon his parents to encourage a process of letting go. One day he was found dead by his family there. He had committed suicide.

For many patients it was impossible to stand on their own two feet. Some of them jumped off the roof when their discharge was announced or tried in some other way to end their lives. A few attempts were successful. For years the patients in Buiten Oord had been able to make social contacts easily. Everything was arranged and done for them. Their free time was planned to be as pleasant as possible, and now suddenly they had to take the big step that for many was too difficult or fatal.

The thought that I would have Raf at home again made me afraid, but there was no other solution. Since Sabina didn't live with me anymore, I could fit up the attic bedroom for Raf. He was by now about 22 years old, and I hoped that living together on two floors would perhaps be more bearable.

But it was soon clear that it was not working

at all without medication. Raf swore to himself, cried, laughed, shrieked, kicked furniture to pieces, and threw coffee cups. He was used to the spaciousness of Buiten Oord where no one had paid attention to him. And because he had felt abandoned by the authorities there, he said that he would never again go to a psychiatrist.

After three weeks of chaos, he turned day into night again. Now I was happy about that, because when he came downstairs at around five o'clock in the afternoon he behaved somewhat calmer. I could now gradually see by small variations in his posture whether a hard day would be in store. Sometimes he had one shoulder hunched up, or one side of his lip hung down somewhat. Then I knew that a relapse might be in the offing. If he didn't feel too ill to receive people, sometimes someone–friends from Buiten Oord— came to visit. One of the boys said that in the meantime he, with a few others, had been to Israel. They had worked in a kibbutz there. But because they couldn't cope with the hard work and the strict discipline, in the end they had to leave.

"Too bad," he said. "You weren't so alone there. The authorities at Buiten Oord had said that we shouldn't hide ourselves away and we should be among other people a lot, but there's a group of us who never go out."

Little by little more reports came out of patients who had been discharged from Buiten Oord. Since they used no medication, some of them went around the city in a dazed state. I heard that a few of them were exploited. They would get some money for carrying little packets. They didn't know what the contents were. Sometimes they came in contact with the law and were taken for drug users and had no defence against that accusation. More and more of them tried to be placed in other institutions.

The picture of Raf's illness, which was now changing all the time, made it impossible for me to get on with things that had to be done. Even working away from home became a problem now that Raf sometimes suddenly behaved so aggressively and started throwing everything around. I got tranquillizers for myself, of which I took full advantage, but I could not go on with them. I decided to phone Dr. van Aken, who had helped Raf before his last hospitalization and whom I hadn't spoken to for at least two years.

"I'll put Raf in touch with the Querido House," he said. "People who have mental problems and aren't yet in a condition to live by themselves are admitted there. They try to teach them a certain adjustment, so that some of them do eventually manage to live on their own. But you'll have to apply directly to the Area Health Authority for the referral."

When I asked for the Department of Mental Hygiene, I got the woman psychiatrist, Mrs. Raas, on the phone again. I hadn't heard her voice for three years, but she must have had a memory like an elephant, for she took up just where she had left off years before.

"So, Mrs. Anstadt, do you think that your

little boy will agree to be admitted to the Querido House?"

"I don't know," I answered nervously.

Does she have to make it still harder for me? I thought. Didn't I already have enough on my plate with Raf at home and a whole clinic-full of former patients around him who kept coming because they were looking for a warm place to sleep?

The day that Raf was summoned to present himself in the Querido House he was in a bad way, but he still wanted to go. He came back in a defiant mood: "I'm not going there," he said. "There are only senile little old men there."

His decision stood firm and I knew that he would not be put off.

"So," said Mrs. Raas when I told her about it. "Can you *still* not get along without your little boy?"

"But Raf cannot be persuaded otherwise," I said.

"In any case, I shall not speak to you any more in the future," she answered. "We have plenty of other things to do than continually being taken up with Raf's situation. You should have put him out on the street, and then he would have had no choice, and *then* he would have gone to the Querido House."

Hadn't I heard that before? "But Raf *is* my son, after all," I said. I still couldn't get used to that harsh approach.

Again I called in the help of Dr. van Aken, who had gradually become my psychiatric advice centre. He promised to send me a social worker. If she could manage to get through to Raf, she could come every week to help him.

On her first visit Raf was lying in bed. He was willing to talk to her. When she came downstairs she said that he had told her a lot. Now she would come every week.

In the meantime it had now become calmer around Raf. His apathy came back, and he also stopped eating and got badly emaciated again. But the social worker couldn't get him to take medication either, so strong was the influence of Buiten Oord on him. We considered what we could do, for the situation was critical.

"You'll have to give him drops in his food," the social worker said. "That's very often done. Raf isn't used to taking tablets, and we won't be able to persuade him to do it willingly in the condition he's in now."

I understood that it had to be done. Raf was also now a danger to himself. Sometimes he lay for hours in front of the fire and had already dropped a burning cigarette on his clothes a couple of times because he had fallen asleep while he was smoking.

Once when I came home from work I smelled a pungent odour of something burning. I ran up the steps. There was nothing on fire in the house as far as I could see. I went to Raf's room, but there was no sign of a fire there, either.

That evening I suddenly missed a big kapok-filled cushion in front of the heater where Raf often lay. Suddenly I understood what must have happened. I went to the porch and found the cushion, soaking wet, with a burnt hole bigger than a football.

When Raf came downstairs that evening to drink something, I asked him what had happened.

"I put the cushion against the heater and fell asleep," he said. "When I woke up I couldn't help coughing a lot, and the room was full of smoke because the cushion was on fire. Then I held it under the tap and put it on the veranda. I opened the window. Before you came home I closed it again."

I took the advice of the social worker and began to put medicines in Raf's food. By this time he had been ill for nearly eight years, and he had been at home and out of Buiten Oord for four months. He apparently needed only a few medicines.

In a week he was speaking in an ordinary way – clearly, no longer incoherently. He was again interested in his surroundings, ate better, and got up early. Now and then he went to neighbours' houses, renewed contacts with friends whom he hadn't seen for a long time, and once more he had visitors. His quick recovery seemed unreal and almost unbelievable.

My house was full again, as it had been before. When I asked Raf to go to his room with his friends, he said, "They don't like the atmosphere there. They just want to stay in the living room because they have no real home. They're always in rented rooms."

Most of them had also become very withdrawn and had nothing to talk about. For that reason, too, they found it safer to stay downstairs with me. I asked questions and talked with them, and they didn't have to give an answer, and that made them feel less isolated and detached.

That was when Raf got to know Eddy. "He's a nice guy. He's just been discharged from the Berg Clinic," Raf explained to me. A couple of days later he came with Raf. I noticed that they had a lot in common and got along well together. Eddy stayed for a meal and came every day after that. He was an intelligent boy and could still concentrate well then.

"What do you say we go to evening classes?" Eddy asked Raf one day. "We really must finish school sometime."

Raf thought it was a good idea. One day after that Eddy had made an appointment with the head, and after an exploratory conversation Raf and he were admitted to the third class of the school.

"How did the headmaster test you?" I asked Raf.

"We were asked some questions that we could both answer easily."

I realized that the headmaster had noticed nothing unusual about them. But it could also be that he wanted to give them a chance because they had remembered so much of their old subjects.

I tried to look at Raf from the point of view

of an outsider. In fact, he looked good. He had now been having drops in his food for two months, and it seemed to me it was as though the difficulties had never existed. I enjoyed this period of relief.

But just as I had feared, things didn't go well at the evening classes. Raf, who had always been an outstanding pupil, didn't once open his books. When I went into his room I saw that some of them were still wrapped in plastic. I got the impression that Raf went to school because he wanted to have the feeling of belonging somewhere. After school he and Eddy, who played the flute, often went with a group to a little café where they talked about music.

Eddy managed to get a few more passing grades, but how Raf could still keep up at school without doing anything for it I didn't understand. When Eddy had another episode within six months and didn't get out of bed any more, neither of them went back.

Raf, who was naturally helpful, went to see Eddy every day, told him stories about the Milky Way, a youth club near the Leidseplein, and took along goodies for him to get him into a better mood. After one of his episodes, which in general didn't last long, Eddy once told me what Raf had done to help him. "I wouldn't have been able to do it," he said. "Sometimes I feel guilty about it. I can't focus on other people like that."

"Oh, you two need each other," I said to put his mind at rest. "Raf helps you because he can't get along without you, either. So it's in his own interest, too."

Raf kept telling everyone that he had a band. Sometimes he even promised people that they could work with him. He spent almost all of the money he had left over from the dole on instruments, which were put in the attic.

"I'm waiting until the band is complete," he would say as an excuse for not being able to use them. If he hadn't acted so strangely in regard to the band, I would have almost forgotten that he was ill.

By now he again had a girlfriend that he had met at the evening classes and who knew nothing about his illness. One day Raf said that he wanted to go to Israel with her. I was shocked. I hadn't wanted to think about that possibility. Then I wouldn't have a chance to administer the medication that he depended on totally. I was certain that without his medicine drops, within a week Raf would again be as sick as before, and I hoped that he wouldn't go through with his plan. But after a few days he began to talk about his passport. He had gone with a tourist pass to Denmark, but now he needed a proper passport. So his intention was serious.

Now I had to tell him the truth. For a while I toyed with the idea that he would perhaps understand that medication was absolutely essential for him. I sought a favourable moment to explain it to him, because I was afraid of his reaction.

The next evening when we were calmly

drinking coffee, I broached the subject. "Raf, now that you want to go to Israel, I must tell you something," I said nervously. "You've noticed that recently things have been going well for you, but..."

"What?" asked Raf.

"For a year now I've been putting medicine drops in your food."

He looked at me without saying anything and blushed. His eyes slowly filled with tears, which kept trickling down his face. He remained quiet for a while. Then he said, "I thought I'd done it myself."

He stood up and went to his room. Only after two days did he come to eat again, and he took food out of the fridge himself.

Now the whole miserable business began again. Raf didn't want to see anyone; he didn't even let Eddy in. He held long incomprehensible conversations with himself. Sometimes I could catch words of it, like...*sad ...manage...not...no...warm sun, where*?... Sometimes he cried while he was talking.

Chapter 8   Saviour of the World

A year passed in which Raf didn't recover. He had a few serious episodes one after the other and then was more confused than before. He got onto trains without paying. All sorts of things happened in different parts of the country. Once the police in Venlo phoned: "Why don't you have your son hospitalized?" they asked.

"My son is 23 years old," I said resignedly. "He doesn't want to be hospitalized."

I got more complaints. I kept having to explain everything and straighten things out. Raf didn't comply with any rules whatsoever. He went to public places without paying. If he was arrested he gave his address and said simply that he hadn't thought about it or that he had forgotten to take money with him. They could see that he was telling the truth and sometimes they let him alone.

His outward appearance was now also changed. He dressed carelessly in loud colours, with scarves around his waist and his neck. His hair was down to his shoulders and in his eyes. He walked slowly, hunched up and shuffling, spoke indistinctly, monotonously, and very softly.

Sometimes I still put some medicine in his food, but I was always afraid that he would notice it. After all those years I had become despondent, sometimes to the point of indifference. I had absolutely no more hope. I was now acutely aware that I would have to bear the difficulties myself. Many more would still come that I would have to be prepared for and for which I would have to find solutions. It concerned my own son, and I now found that I couldn't imagine anyone else being responsible for him.

A resignation set in that at the same time also gave me some strength. When I went home from work I took Librium to shore up my courage and to keep Raf from feeling that his illness gave me so much trouble. He quickly noticed how anyone was feeling and suffered from it when I was sad. I wanted to try to give a little colour to the unhappy life that he led.

After the year in which Raf had caused more and more problems, there was suddenly a lull. I realised only after some time that nothing spectacular was happening any more with him and that he only rarely left the house. Now another pattern became increasingly apparent. He could go from a turbulent, restless urge to roam to complete apathy in which he no longer did anything and hallucinated a lot. For a long time I no longer invited my own friends over. Only disturbed acquaintances of Raf's sometimes still came – if he let them in, that is.

Sabina also sometimes came. She was still the easiest person for Raf to talk to, because she got along with him in an easy-going way now that she was used to him. But she lived at the edge of the city and had her own problems that demanded her attention.

I tried with all my might to keep our life bearable. When Raf felt well I sometimes asked him to play chess with me. Sometimes he was willing to play and then looked so sorrowful and embarrassed, as though he were saying: "That's all that's left for me, and you've figured me out." Yet he played well.

In the weekends I would suggest baking cakes, or I would ask him to help me prepare the meal. Something had to be done to activate him because there was less life in him by the day.

When I talked to my psychiatrist, he said, "You must be prepared for Raf needing you less and less. When his hallucinations engross him deeply and he hears many voices, he would rather stay in that world. That doesn't mean that you mustn't try to get him out of it. It is important that he is also still involved with the outside world, for hallucinatory images frighten the sick person, and he is sometimes thankful to be distracted from them."

That winter Eddy also had a serious psychotic episode. His mother was at the end of her tether and called up Raf to ask, "Will you try and see whether Eddy will let you in? For days now he has had his door locked and he's run out of food."

Raf indeed seemed to be the only one who got entrance to Eddy's room. This task revived Raf a bit and made him feel that he was again needed somewhere. He went every day to his friend and also took him hot food. He told me that Eddy was in a bad way but didn't share any details.

In the evening I heard him mumbling to himself, "That can't go on like that." But when I asked what couldn't go on, he didn't answer. I got the feeling that he found it indelicate to talk about their illnesses and thought that their troubles should stay within their circle, because only insiders could understand them.

After a week Eddy's mother called again. She said that neighbourhood boys had found her son on the ice-cold floor of his room. Eddy had thrown everything out of the window, including his bed. That same night he was taken to the Berg Clinic again. The boys who had notified her had taken Eddy's TV set and blamed Raf for the theft. The mother had understood the situation.

Raf was upset by the hospitalization of his friend. After two weeks he went to visit him, but Eddy didn't recognize him. Raf cried when he came home.

Raf was not very concerned about money. Out of the benefit he received he gave me what I asked for as a contribution to household expenses, but beyond that he found it unimportant. He spent very little. Of late he had also stopped buying musical instruments, and that increased his savings. He regularly made withdrawals from his giro account, and if someone in the street held out his hand, he gave him everything he had. He himself needed nothing, he said. When he was going around with Eddy, Eddy had restrained him from giving his money away. They had had a corrective influence on each other. Now it had happened twice recently that Raf had given someone a 100-guilder note. The first time it happened he came home and asked me, "Mum, give me 10 guilders. I've run out."

"But this morning you still had so much money," I said, surprised.

"Well, there was a woman with a baby on the Dam Square who needed it."

I gave him money in the hope that this would be a one-off, but when the same thing happened shortly afterwards, I explained to him that what he was giving was too much.

He said that in future he would carry no more than 10 guilders. But this still led to other problems. One evening he went out and came home at ten o'clock (whereas he had recently been staying out half the night), so I asked him what the matter was.

"Ten guilders is too little," he answered, resigned and smiling.

"How's that?"

"In a café a guy wanted to have a beer off me, and when I said I didn't have any more money he took a gun out of his pocket. I put my wallet on the bar and left."

He said that he hadn't been afraid. That didn't surprise me. Raf did everything in the same calm tempo, in complete faith that nothing could happen to him. I had a strong suspicion that he still laboured under the delusion that he was Jesus Christ.

After the incident in that café he carried 25 guilders with him. Sometimes he bought hand-made things for me in the community centre and, as second-hand clothing was sold there, he occasionally bought something for himself. Latterly he didn't spend any more than that.

For that reason it alarmed me when he had left his giro accounts lying about and I saw that twice in one week he had withdrawn 500 guilders. I was afraid that now he had come in contact with drugs and asked him what he had done with all that money. He didn't answer.

That evening he carried on an intense conversation with himself. Sometimes I could break up this sort of conversation if I demanded his attention, but if he spoke with such deep concentration in himself as he was doing now, I couldn't do it. He waved me away and cupped his hand to his ear so as to be able to listen to himself better.

"You mustn't do that," I heard him say. "You look so sweet and you're so young. You make me unhappy."

He spoke very tenderly with someone, and I wanted to know more about it. "Who makes you unhappy?" I asked. His conversation switched over to me.

"If I can't sleep I sometimes go walking around in the neighbourhood at night. I've noticed that there are a lot of little prostitutes living here in the side street. Sometimes I talk to them. But I didn't know that some of those very young girls were also prostitutes. This week I went upstairs with one of them. I told her that she looked so sweet and that she mustn't do that any more. I asked if she would promise that. I had just got 500 guilders from the bank. I gave it to her with my crown. I said that she must keep it safely. Look, I have another one."

He showed me a shiny label with a golden crown on it from some shop or other with a royal warrant.

"But then what did you do with the second 500 guilders?"

"The next evening I went past her house. She was standing there again and she wanted to have the money again."

My psychiatrist, whose help I enlisted for this new problem, explained to me that these ideas clearly fitted in with Raf's illness. "I remember," he said, "that you said years ago that Raf wanted to be a 'rescuing figure' and that for a while he imagined that he was Jesus Christ. His delusions of grandeur have developed by degrees.

"First he was the hero from the books of Karl May, then the world-famous singer Bob Dylan, and finally Jesus Christ himself. It is clear that he now also feels himself to be a kind of saviour of the world. Delusions of grandeur often present in schizophrenics in the canonization of prostitutes, whereby the women's virginity is restored. When Raf sees that girl who is offering herself for sale, he doesn't understand that such sweet girls are prostitutes and he gives her not only his money but also his crown. From that it would appear that he thinks that he possesses superhuman powers with which he can restore her innocence.

"These delusions of grandeur can become increasingly comprehensive and then manifest themselves as thoughts of being omnipotent. But the schizophrenic is also sometimes consumed by great anxieties that he tries to escape in his world of imagination.

"He also knows moments of bliss in which he is visited by visions of redemption, a feeling of happiness that can be very deep. It is striking that those blissful visions often resemble those of other schizophrenics.

"The visions in the delusions have clear patterns. They are related to the dream visions and images received through prayer, which in other cultures are regarded as divine revelations. Almost always God and the devil are involved in them. The devil is a terrifying element, God is the conciliatory figure. For the sick person the devil is the enemy, the adversary. God is not only the ally who offers help, but also the gestalt of the patient himself. God and the schizophrenic become one. This union can produce a deep blissfulness. God manifests himself sometimes also as the Christ bringing peace or as a radiant figure on his throne in heaven. The devil is often a goat-like half-human with horns, like something left over from medieval legends. You could say that the schizophrenic reproduces these figures as symbols of the struggle between good and evil in him. This explanation of the theory isn't much help to you. You can't help Raf. The best thing would be for him to have himself hospitalized again."

But Raf didn't consider it. He now frequently went to the youth club in the city and brought people with him to his room late at night. I generally had to send them away, because they played loud music. When I went upstairs, I noticed that Raf usually slept through the racket. Once when I found it too awful I woke him up. In contrast to the beginning of his illness, I had learned to treat him calmly in all circumstances. Veiled aggression or anger on my part he sensed keenly and it confused him. Then he could sometimes look at me with a determined expression and a furious look in his eyes without saying anything. In a situation like that it was not possible to have a conversation with him.

In those years of his illness I had learned by experience that I could talk to him only in an easy-going way. "Raf," I said, "you can't bring people home so late. We can't do that to our neighbours."

"They always want to come along," he said resignedly, "even if I don't want them to. Just send them away."

Once twelve fellows all came at the same time in the middle of the night. When I went upstairs I saw that Raf was nervous. He wanted them to go away, but evidently the word had got round that you could sleep in Raf's room. He couldn't cope with so many people and was amazed that I did manage to get rid of them.

"I'm giving you fifteen minutes to get out of here," I said, "or else I'm calling the police. I want to keep living in my house and I don't want to get thrown out of it because of your doing." They went. It struck me that they didn't make any trouble and seemed to appreciate my arguments.

Another time, when Raf didn't get up in the

morning, I heard a dog bark in his room. Through a big crack in his door I saw someone lying on the floor with a hypodermic syringe beside him. A dog on a rope lay up against him.

The animal began to growl. I called through the crack, "Will you please go away within half an hour."

When I went upstairs later the man had disappeared – in great haste, as I noticed, for the hypodermic syringe still lay there and the floor was strewn with coins.

In those days there were not yet so many drug addicts going about in the city, and the few that there were wanted to keep a low profile.

"That man had asked in such a pathetic way if he could just once sleep in my warm room, too" Raf said later. "And his dog looked so sad. I didn't know that he was a junkie. I went straight to sleep."

"But when you saw that needle?" I asked.

"I didn't see it until you said that he had to leave."

Now I couldn't sleep peacefully at night. I had always managed to get rid of the people, but now I lay awake for hours, because since the visit from that junkie I expected disturbers of the peace who were still more unsavoury.

After that time Raf seldom brought more than one person home with him.

My psychiatrist said that Raf was afraid of his hallucinatory images and so didn't want to be alone. Lately girls had come along, too, whom I then met in the morning downstairs in the hallway because they also used my shower, sometimes so lavishly that I had to go to work without having a shower myself. There were also foreign girls who in this way had a cheap place to stay overnight.

Once Raf had brought along a German girl. That morning I heard from him that he was going with her to Germany. He came back again that same evening. In North Brabant they had visited a couple of her friends. "They wanted to have money from me," Raf said. "I thought they had a nerve, because before that time I had already given that girl 200 guilders. I wasn't going to get ripped off like that. When I didn't give them anything, they started a fight. I got so furious that I fought back hard and then I left." He added, laughing, "I don't think they expected me to be so strong."

He behaved very lucidly, clearly shaken awake by this experience.

I discussed the latest events with my brother. "Let Raf come and stay with us for a month," he said. "Then you can have some peace and quiet. I'll put it to Raf that it's for the sake of your health. Then he'll be sure to agree."

"Then try to put some medicine in his food again. He won't expect it from you," I said.

But when Raf was with my brother, it turned out that he no longer reacted well to his medicines. Perhaps it also happened because it wasn't very restful there. My brother always had a house full of people because his wife felt herself called upon to help everyone who was having a rough time. Raf fell in love with a girl who went to visit regularly and who brushed aside his advances. A young man from Canada also lived there who drank a lot and got Raf out of bed at night because he wanted to go to bars with him.

When Raf came back I made an appointment with his psychiatrist, who spoke first with Raf and then with me.

"The medicines that he was given still work," he said. "But Raf has now been ill for more than ten years. You'll have to give him more. I think he also ought to have something else in addition, because he acted very dejected at our appointment. Perhaps we can change something there. You should now mix his drops with a powder and put it in the jam on his bread. If that doesn't work, try it in the evening in the pudding, or something else that's sweet."

Because I looked startled, he emphasised his words: "Mrs. Anstadt, I understand that you hate the idea, but as long as he refuses to go into hospital that's the only thing that can help Raf and you a bit."

In the first days I managed to give Raf his medicine, and sure enough he quickly became less groggy. He was obviously in better spirits.

We were sitting talking one morning when he suddenly went to his room and a half hour later came back with a holdall filled with the essential things for a trip. He said that he felt well and wanted to go away for a little while. I was shocked but I controlled myself. I had already seen at breakfast a far, strange gleam in his eyes. It had made me sad because I thought I had detected something of a fresh, new spirit in him. I was disappointed that he had only just got his new medicines and now they had to be stopped again. I knew from experience how this urge to roam would turn out. He would, as always, come home dazed and filthy and not remember anything of this project. I also knew that there was absolutely no point in my opposing him.

When Raf was away my anxiety gave way to a feeling of resignation. I recalled that I myself hadn't been on a trip for a long time either and decided to make use of this situation to have a holiday.

I wanted to try not to worry about all the difficulties that awaited me until after my return. I joined some friends who were making a trip through Italy and enjoyed this carefree time so much that I was even very cheerful. But the nearer my return to Amsterdam came, the more nervous I got.

When I went into my house my worry seemed not to have been unfounded. Raf couldn't persevere for very long in being away from home and considering that, he must have been back for quite a while. The whole house looked as though rubbish bins had been overturned in every room. It was a warm day and the smell was unbearable. Raf was in his underpants and was wearing blue sunglasses without lenses and had on a cloth cap that he often wore when he was having an episode of mental illness.

On the sofa in my room a young fellow lay sleeping. I shuddered when I looked at him. He looked filthy and his feet were so black they looked as if they could never be clean again. It looked as though his skin had absorbed the black colour into itself. I had apparently disturbed him, for he woke up. He said nothing, stood up, went to the hallway, put on his jacket, and disappeared without saying a word to me.

I tried to explain to Raf that I found this mess outrageous. But he just chuckled and was in no state to have a normal conversation.

"Raf, won't you at least put some clothes on?" I asked. "Please, try to come to your senses a bit. You must help me clear up this mess".

He looked at me somewhat more attentively, probably because my voice trembled from suppressed tears, and he stopped chuckling. He took the cap off, disappeared to his room, and came downstairs a little later to take a shower. I saw that he was going through the pockets of his jacket that hung on the hall stand. Suddenly he said in a completely normal voice, "That guy's pinched my wallet with 100 guilders in it."

As usual when something serious had happened he became lucid, but also sad and quiet. "Why does a guy like that do that, anyway?" he said with a mournful tone. "He was here for days and I didn't even know him."

"Exactly," I answered. "You'll have to learn to understand that not everyone is nice. Try to be a bit more careful. Really, Raf, you can't trust everyone."

Because he was roaming around a lot again these days I could give him medicine only infrequently. It became more and more obvious that he would have to be hospitalized. The older he got the worse his illness became.

Dr. van Aken said that it was necessary to start Raf on new medication. It was obvious to everyone how disturbed he was. He went through the streets in strange clothing gesticulating and talking loudly to himself. He had also now adopted a peculiar manner. He held one arm bent and let his hand hang limply with the palm downward. For days he walked around like that, like a dog offering its paw. I tried once to say something about it, but I noticed that it meant more to him than I could guess. He first looked menacingly at me and then at his hand that seemed to behave independently of him, like a foreign object. When he then looked up at me again, I saw a frightened and at the same time a somewhat imploring expression in his eyes. I understood that his hand for one reason or another must stay like that and that something depended on it that he couldn't explain to me. My remark had apparently confused him.

When I talked about it with the psychiatrist later, he said, "It's better that you just let him go in his compulsive behaviour. Probably he mustn't let the hand be lowered. He may imagine that much depends on it."

Raf was now also having problems in the street. Gradually more drug users had come into Amsterdam. People thought that he, too, was an addict and became less friendly to him, whereas earlier they had behaved more helpfully and indulgently.

Once when I was walking with a friend in the street we bumped into Raf. He looked less confused than usual but more discouraged. "I'm not allowed into that café any more." He gestured with his head toward the other side of the street. "There's a new owner. The old one was so nice. Everybody I know is there. I haven't done anything, either."

The more confused he became the more often he set himself tasks that he couldn't cope with.

He went to do a nightshift at the post office. There they very often took on odd characters, but the next morning Raf was sent home with one day's pay. He didn't understand why he had been dismissed. He didn't know that he kept talking to himself while he was working and then did nothing because he was at that moment in another world that had nothing in common with his surroundings. He began to work again only when he was urged to. After such a dismissal he was ashamed and became still more depressed because of it. He wanted so much to persevere and he always had setbacks.

I didn't see him downstairs again for days then, and his condition, in which he didn't eat and hallucinated a lot, got more serious by the day. Finally I advised him not to go to work. I said that the weather was too beautiful and that he could better go walking in the Vondel Park. But then he looked at me so incredulously with wide-open eyes that I was ashamed of my transparent game.

He was allowed to work for a while for the mother of a girlfriend that he knew from the institution. She made paper flowers. But quite quickly he learned that he might go and talk, but that he could work only one afternoon a week.

"Why can't I work every day?" he asked me. "I like the work."

"Maybe, in the end, she didn't have enough work for herself," I answered, "and so she would rather make the flowers just with her daughter."

He was not yet sick enough to be able to come to terms with the fact that he was in the way everywhere. I could hardly bear his isolation, and sometimes I hoped that he would get into a situation that he would find unendurable. He now often sat for hours in a corner of the living room, quiet, with a sorrowful expression and with his head down, as though he was wondering what he was to do with his life, such as it was. I couldn't help him at all. He got totally withdrawn into himself, and I was happy that I had work that enabled me to extricate myself from this stress for a part of the day.

I wasn't surprised when the Crisis Centre of the Wilhemina Gasthuis, of which Raf's psychiatrist had in the meantime become director, phoned me one day. "Mrs. Anstadt," he said, "Raf has come here and says that he isn't leaving again. He's too incoherent for a conversation, but he must have had the feeling that he couldn't go on like this. Don't worry. We won't send him away. I'll wait until he calms down and then I'll try to find out whether he wants to be admitted to an institution again."

After a few days it was decided that if Raf would agree to hospitalization he would go to the Berg Clinic, where the patients were treated with medicines. I was happy with this choice, because I wanted no more alternative institutions.

After two weeks I heard that Raf had consented to be admitted to the Berg Clinic.

Chapter 9 Heleen

On my first visit I saw that he was enjoying the pleasant atmosphere and the well-kept interior there. He also told me about the religious holidays that were celebrated. He was interested and so he happily took part in them. Religious and mystical things had held a special attraction for him for a long time.

We went walking in the woods and Raf was noticeably talkative. The new surroundings had made him somewhat more lucid. He told me about the strict discipline in the Clinic. "I think that's a good idea," he said.

I remembered that even as a child he had liked to keep to strict rules. In this period of his illness he had repeatedly done his best to get out of the house and not sleep all day, much as he often didn't relish the idea. The trips that he made from time to time and that he sometimes managed for only a few days were also evidence that he repeatedly tried to triumph over himself. I sometimes thought that this self-discipline and the demands that he placed on himself would help slow down the process of his decline, which was like a river silting up. With his remaining intellectual abilities he did his very best to keep up.

"I play chess a lot," he said. "There are good chess players here, so I have to try really hard to win." He looked contented. "I'll stay here until I feel well enough to go to work."

I went to visit him regularly, and he said

that he got few medicines. "At first I didn't want to have any pills at all. But I have a strict psychiatrist and he said that it was required here. When I feel better I want to take the entrance examination for the Music Lyceum. I've already talked about it with the psychiatrist here. He likes the idea."

Because after all those years I knew from experience that this recovery of Raf's would be of a temporary nature, his new plan frightened me. I wondered if the psychiatrist would really let him experience this disappointment. Latterly Raf had not once been in a state to read through a whole piece of music. But he seemed to have persevered; he had filled in the forms. When a letter for him came to my address from the Music Lyceum saying that he had to sit the exam on a certain day, I phoned his psychiatrist.

"We surely can't do that to him," I said anxiously.

"I wouldn't know what to do to prevent it," the psychiatrist answered. "It will be a blow for him, but he thinks he's so terrific in the field of music that he won't believe me if I stop him. So there's nothing much else for it than to wait and see what happens."

Raf told me what he was practising. There was also a Beatles song. I was terror-stricken. I wondered if I should phone the Music Lyceum. I didn't do it. But as it later turned out, they had understood that Raf was ill. After his exam, which had left him dissatisfied, I got a message in which I was informed that the letter was intended for me personally. I had to decide myself how I should discuss it with Raf. Raf was indeed musical, they wrote, but a sick young man. He should, at best, still be able to go to an ordinary music school when he felt better again. I told his psychiatrist, who promised me to pass it on to Raf as carefully as possible.

Raf *was* disappointed but took it all rather more calmly than I had expected. He had now been in the Berg Clinic for four months and felt fairly well. I had already heard that they gave their chronic patients injections with long-lasting effects and then sent them home. They could come to talk at the Bureau for Mental Health Assistance in Amsterdam at regular times and get new injections.

One afternoon Raf suddenly came home upset. He rushed through the rooms as if someone were chasing him.

"Now, calm down. What's happened?" I asked.

"No, I can't calm down," he answered. "I don't know what the doctor's done. I don't know what's happened." He raced around – around the table, through the hallway, in and out of all the rooms.

"I have to choose," he said while he was running. "I've got to do it."

"What do you have to choose?"

"The psychiatrist wanted to give me an injection. Then for three weeks I wouldn't have to take any medicine."

While he was talking he sat down, jumped up again, walked around some more, lay down on the sofa, and stood up again. He couldn't be still for a moment.

"I didn't want any injections," he continued. "Then the psychiatrist said that if I refused injections, I would have to leave immediately. I didn't know what to do. Then I just agreed to it. But I'm afraid. Something's happened." He went to my bedroom, got into my bed, but at once got up again.

"I can't lie still. What can I do?" he asked desperately. "I can't get rid of this agitated feeling. I'll just go and see if I can sleep in my own room."

He went upstairs and was back downstairs within two minutes. Now he was crying, but I noticed that it didn't give him any relief from the stress. I had never experienced this before and felt helpless. I called Hans, who came from The Hague within an hour. Raf had run around all that time like a mad dog without stopping. When Hans got there I phoned the Area Health Authority, because we were afraid that Raf had been given the wrong injection. But the Area Health Authority stayed out of it. They said that they couldn't help and that it did very often happen that some patients had a strong motor reaction to slow-release medication that was administered in large amounts to be gradually absorbed by the body, in which case the medicine was active sometimes for as much as a month.

Hans and I were watching dismayed at how Raf, who was exhausted, kept dashing through the house.

Finally he couldn't stand it there either and

wanted to go back to the Clinic. Hans took him away and I was relieved because I expected that there, at least, they would give him something to make him calmer.

That same evening Raf came back to Amsterdam. He hadn't been able to stand it in the Clinic, either, and had run away from there. Tired from the rushing about, he had finally hailed a taxi and had himself brought to Amsterdam. We watched despairingly as he squirmed and didn't know what to do with himself. Hans finally took him to the Clinic for the second time.

After a week Raf gradually got better. But when, after the agreed-upon three weeks, the psychiatrist came to him again with a hypodermic needle, Raf refused and had to leave. He came home disappointed. He hadn't wanted to leave, but was too frightened of the effects of a new jab.

A few years later the psychiatrist H. M. van Praag wrote that large amounts of medicine had initially been administered to psychiatric patients because it was thought thereby to achieve a better result. But the patients often reacted to it with great anxiety and also sometimes with severe motor disturbances. Each patient seemed to have a different tolerance in relation to medicines. In clinics nowadays, he wrote, it was recommended to take the greatest possible care to ascertain which dose of medicine would yield the best results.

Raf remained at home quiet, listless and distant. This hope of recovery, and all the good intentions that went with it, had also disappeared.

He stayed depressed and gave the impression of being exhausted from the battle. A long time went by when little happened. Raf slept most of the time. Sometimes I still managed to put some medicine in his food that I got from the psychiatrist of the Berg Clinic when he held a surgery in Amsterdam.

Raf now seemed afraid to be alone in his room and took to sleeping in his old nursery, except when he had summoned up the courage to go out and would bring someone from the club to stay with him.

One morning, when he had been sleeping upstairs for a few days, to my amazement he asked, "May a girlfriend of mine take a shower? She's afraid to come downstairs without your permission. She's a bit shy."

That last part reassured me. She came downstairs and behaved more discreetly than I was ever used to from Raf's friends.

That girl began to settle into our house in a quiet, polite manner, without my being able to do anything to oppose it. She greeted me modestly when I met her and I saw that she brought along baskets full of goodies for Raf, who still always stayed in his bed.

Sometimes before I went to work I would have to go upstairs to leave a message for Raf, and I would see that she was reading aloud to him. She looked intelligent and friendly and I didn't understand why she sought out Raf's company.

From time to time a conversation would develop between us when she was in the kitchen.

I couldn't resist asking why she felt attracted to Raf. She said that she would like to help him. She was sweet and calm, just the sort of girl that Raf liked. In his isolation and apathy he was glad to be helped.

Heleen said that she was a kindergarten teacher but that, at the moment, she was unemployed. I was amazed at how patiently she would explain something to Raf when he didn't understand it. She often laid her head on his shoulder and was affectionate toward him. Then he treated her very tenderly, too.

During his illness he often had girlfriends, but in recent years he never spoke to me about his relationships with women. I did know that girls liked him even when he was very confused. Sometimes they phoned. If I liked the sound of their voice and Raf felt too sick to come to the telephone, I would get into a conversation with them. Then I would hear that they found him such a sad, friendly fellow and were eager to help to cheer him up. I had the impression that Raf found all that phoning bothersome. I think that he wanted to be left in peace and wanted to decide on his friends and acquaintances himself.

After some weeks I began to get used to Heleen as a member of the household. She behaved so calmly that I felt at ease in her company.

In one of our conversations I asked her if she herself had a house.

"I've lived in a commune," she said. "Near

Maastricht. It was great there. Sometimes I long to go back. But I want to try to find a job here and I'm probably getting a house from my mother. She has a couple of little houses and something is going to be free shortly. My sister, who lives there, is going to move in with her boyfriend. Raf wants to come with me."

That seemed to me a safe option; Raf under Heleen's wing. I did wonder again how he would get his medicine. But I couldn't very well chain him to myself all my life. On the other hand, I knew for sure that in the long run Heleen wouldn't be able to stand him without medicine, either. I toyed with the idea of taking her into my confidence.

Now she came more and more often into the kitchen or into the living room to talk when Raf was sleeping. Sometimes he came too. I believe that this time was especially pleasant for all three of us.

It was striking how they resembled each other, in their appearance as well as in their behaviour. They both had dark eyes and dark hair and behaved in a friendly and calm manner. They spoke in an easy-going way to each other. I noticed that Raf felt better by the day because of Heleen's presence.

Gradually Heleen got to know our family and circle of friends. She was accepted by everyone and also got to be friends with Sabina. They were of the same age and both liked to draw. But it remained a puzzle what she saw in Raf. Hans also asked her what bound her to Raf, but her answers were always evasive.

She had a great interest in many areas and could talk about them at length with Hans as well as Sabina's husband, for she was by now married. In the afternoon when I wasn't working Heleen and Raf sometimes came downstairs. Heleen would embroider or draw and Raf would sit still and look at her without doing anything, but looking more contented than I had seen him in years. Heleen often made tea for us, cooked tasty things, and tried to make the place welcoming. Sometimes a conversation developed in which Raf also took part, drawn out of his isolation because something had caught his interest and taken him away from his troubles.

Now and then Heleen and I went to a pavement café or to a museum when Raf didn't feel like going out. It was as if I had known her for years. But I still noticed that she didn't like to talk to me about Raf. She accepted him as he was and had only a tender expression when I tried to bring up a problem that involved him.

After six months they were going to move. I expected that it would all go well. Raf was behaving in a more balanced way, didn't talk to himself much, and didn't hallucinate noticeably. He was still very quiet and didn't laugh much. But when they had moved, it seemed that Raf had a need to come and drink coffee with me every day. Not only was that companionable but it also solved the problem of the medicine for the time being. After a week, when they had got their own house in order, Raf and Heleen asked me to come for a meal. I knew that Heleen never cooked and ate very little. But when I was with them it seemed that Raf, who used to be a good cook, had done his best.

Their little house consisted of half a dwelling: a room about five metres square and a little kitchen. Everything was already there, and they didn't have to buy anything.

It was summertime. They often went walking for hours and came tired and contented to visit me. Raf now went with Heleen again to the youth club. One evening he met a fellow there whom he hadn't seen for a long time and had first met at Eddy's. Harry, who during a trip to Israel was arrested because of his aggressive behaviour, said that he was now discharged from the clinic where Eddy was still being cared for. He said that Eddy was in a really bad way.

Raf once came with Harry to visit me. I found him agitated, aggressive and overbearing. I asked Raf not to bring him to my house again.

Harry, who reminded Raf of his imaginary "band", came to him every day with new plans.

"We're going to start a new group," Raf said. "And Harry thinks that I need to buy another guitar. The one I have he doesn't think is good enough."

"Do you think it's not good enough either?" I asked.

"Oh, I'd be glad to have a better one. For our band we need an electric one."

They got all worked up about hare-brained

schemes that I knew made no sense and would only end in disappointment.

Heleen played the piano well, but she didn't like Harry either and kept quiet and aloof in the hope that all these plans they were making would blow over.

But from one day to the next Harry got Raf more and more in his power, and Raf became more and more out of touch with reality because of all the fantasy about the future. Harry now also frequently took him with him and Heleen stayed at home alone. Raf and Heleen still came regularly to see me in the afternoon, but Raf now behaved less calmly. Often he said to her, "Would you mind staying with my mother? I have to go to the rehearsal."

When he went away Heleen sometimes took up a book or drew something. She wasn't willing to talk about their recent difficulties.

Gradually, Harry also began coming to their house in the middle of the night and even got into the habit of taking acquaintances there who had no place to sleep. Once Raf and Heleen had a little disagreement about it while I was present. Heleen couldn't stand all the commotion but was no match for Harry with his tyrannical behaviour.

She became noticeably quiet and thin. Her eyes were big and she looked frightened. I couldn't help them and it was clear that Raf was spoiling their relationship by doing this. He didn't see it yet, so wrapped up was he with his nonexistent band.

On one of the afternoons at home with me I

noticed that Heleen was behaving differently than usual. She was excited, upset, even aggressive, and talked constantly. There was no stopping her.

Raf looked at her silently. When she became a bit calmer he asked her in a concerned tone of voice, "Has it done you some good to get it off your chest?"

And to me: "At home she almost never says anything any more, and she doesn't eat either, whatever I cook." Although he was seriously concerned, he didn't make the connection with the problem about Harry.

When they had gone away a vague fear came over me. I had noticed by Heleen's behaviour recently that in their negative words she and Raf both reacted in the same way. Her withdrawn behaviour, the fact that she didn't eat, and the strange, aggressive way in which she could suddenly express herself, made me think of Raf when he couldn't cope with a situation.

But they kept coming every afternoon, both of them silent and in a depressed mood. Heleen looked very bad. Her eyes, which had always looked so friendly, were now glassy from fear. I had the impression that they kept coming to get support in their difficulties. But I knew that I would not be able to get Raf to break off the friendship with Harry, and as long as Heleen wasn't able to tell Raf what was bothering her, nothing would change.

Raf was very concerned about her and suggested going to the South of France for a little while. Maybe that would do her good. Heleen got slightly better, probably from the prospect of a break. I was now concerned about both of them. I was afraid that something would happen to Heleen abroad and that Raf wouldn't be able to cope with the situation, certainly not without medicine. They went off in a reasonable frame of mind with the Magic Bus and the least possible amount of baggage. They planned to stay until Heleen felt better.

But after a week they were back. "It was so quiet there," said Heleen. "We didn't have anybody to talk to all day long."

"We were homesick for Holland," said Raf. "Heleen wanted to come back to go to the club at night and to talk with you."

As soon as Harry knew that they were back in the country he took up all Raf's time, just as before, and Heleen became still quieter.

The weekend after their return Heleen and Raf went to his father's family in The Hague. They had already made this arrangement previously. Before they left they came over for a little while. Raf looked serious. I gathered something had happened that he didn't want to talk about, and that he was afraid that something would go wrong.

Heleen was shaking as though she were cold. She looked pale, but in spite of her uneasiness willingly let herself be led. She knew Hans and his family well and liked them.

That same evening Hans phoned me. His voice sounded worried. "The meal was tough going," he said. "Heleen made the atmosphere so gloomy that we finished up the meal quickly. I think she's sick. She's gone back to Amsterdam in a seriously depressed state."

The next day Heleen came over without Raf. I had the impression that she was at the end of her tether. "I'm coping worse and worse with my melancholy," she said.

She began with a soft voice on a story that she probably had wanted to tell for a long time. "When I came to Raf last year, I had already spent a year in a psychiatric institution near Breda. I was discharged as completely cured and didn't have to take any more medicine. The psychiatrist did advise me to avoid stressful situations, though. In the beginning it was calm and relaxed with Raf."

"Was that your first hospitalization?" I asked.

"No," she answered. "Two years before that, after I had passed my headmistress certificate and had worked too hard, I was hospitalized for the first time. I had to promise the psychiatrist at the institution to get in touch with him as soon as I felt that it was necessary."

"And so are you going to do that?" I asked worriedly. "Aren't you waiting too long?"

She hung her head, but then looked at me with a knowing glance and nodded. She understood that I knew that any minute now it could be too late. As soon as she was confused she would forget all about her agreement with her psychiatrist.

Raf had been with Harry and when he came to collect Heleen, she burst out furiously at him for the first time. It pained me to see how clumsily she did that. But now that everything had become too much for her, she lost control of herself and she was for the first time in a state to tell Raf what she thought of the situation. Finally she said that she couldn't stand Harry, that Raf was always abandoning her for him and the band, and that she couldn't bear the situation any longer. It all came out in stammering.

Raf looked unhappy and said to me, "It's so unpleasant at home now. I'll have to go away. Heleen never says a word." For a while I had been struck by the fact that he talked about her and not to her.

Before they left I asked Heleen again to promise me to get in touch with her psychiatrist as quickly as possible.

After that I heard nothing from them for a couple of days. After a week I became worried and went to see them.

Heleen lay in bed. She reacted in such a dazed way that a conversation seemed no longer possible. But it gave me a still greater shock that Raf also now seemed to be in a psychotic state. He didn't react to my arrival and was busy with a thick felt-tipped marker writing all over the walls strange words like "Hilifi", "Malafa", and "Abalafa". I remembered this state of his. He had very often scribbled incomprehensible words all over the walls. The situation with Heleen had probably become too much for him.

I made tea and served sandwiches. Then I said, "Raf, you do understand that something has got to happen, don't you? You two can't stay here like this."

He looked at me despairingly and then said to Heleen, "You can't go away. You can't let them take you in. Do you hear, Heleen? You mustn't go into hospital. I'll take good care of you."

Then he turned his gaze on me again as though I would be able to come to his rescue. But as long as she herself didn't give permission for hospital admittance, I could not ask the Area Health Authority for help. I could, therefore, for the time being do nothing and went away with the realization that the situation would have to get still worse before measures could be taken.

That same night Raf phoned me again. "Will you please come?' Heleen's getting worse and worse. I don't know what to do."

I immediately took a taxi. When I got there I gave Heleen a Valium tablet to make her calmer, because she was talking gibberish. She quickly fell asleep. Raf also went to sleep quickly, exhausted by the events.

I phoned the Mental Hygiene Department of the Area Health Authority.

The psychiatrist didn't come until the middle of the next day. "I advise you to go to Accidents and Emergencies with her," he said, "because in Pavilion Three there's no room for an immediate admittance."

"But my son is also disturbed by this situation and is also in an acute psychosis. They are friends and live together, and so there must be a way for that girl to be admitted. I can't leave them alone in this state. I have to go to work."

135

"I understand," he answered. "But I don't know any solution for you."

I phoned for a taxi. Heleen murmured some unintelligible sentences but went along without resisting. Raf was still asleep.

In the waiting room in Accidents and Emergencies I laid Heleen on the wooden bench and covered her with her coat, in which she wrapped herself up like a baby. She stuck her finger in her mouth and muttered something.

We waited there for hours. There was no psychiatrist free to see me.

In the meantime Raf had woken up toward evening. When he saw that we weren't at home he went to look for us everywhere and finally ended up at Accidents and Emergencies, too. By now it had become eleven o'clock. Raf began to cry when he saw us and kept repeating that Heleen must not be hospitalized.

The noise that we were making was perhaps an unusual symptom for the A and E department. Heleen, her hair in a tangle, looked around sleepily. She didn't understand what the matter was. In any case, someone now came to have a look. Very shortly after that a woman psychiatrist arrived. She looked at me for a moment without saying anything.

I had used the hours in the waiting room to keep Heleen calm and had had no time to think about it all. The psychiatrist looked at Raf and at Heleen and then at me and said, "This can't go on like this. You can't possibly handle this yourself. That girl must be admitted at once."

136

Raf looked at us with anxious eyes, took Heleen, who was uninvolved in it herself, by the hand and ran away with her.

I had been taken up with her for 24 hours, was dead tired, and could barely still react. The psychiatrist stayed sitting with me for a while and wordlessly put her arm around me. This gesture brought me back to myself.

"You must phone me the moment your son and his girlfriend agree to be admitted. Whatever happens, there will be room for her. It's an impossible job for you to take on the responsibility for two psychotic patients."

The next night Raf phoned me. He was afraid of Heleen. "Mum, you have to come and get her," he said. "I don't want to stay at home any more. This Heleen has become so different."

I tried to calm him down and said that I would come right away but that he mustn't leave before I got there. When I came, Raf lay down on the floor and in a moment fell asleep exhausted. I saw that in the meantime the walls had been written over even more, now with ladders drawn through everything. Between every rung there was a number. Also in places that were still free of writing Raf had put the name "Hilifi" with a red marker.

Heleen walked back and forth, got into bed, got up again, straightened the blankets, and got into bed again. She talked to herself non-stop in unintelligible sentences.

I gave her some Valium again, stayed awake the whole night, and when I phoned the

Wilhelmina Gasthuis the next morning I was quickly put through to the psychiatrist whom I had spoken to the previous evening.

On the way to Pavilion Three Raf comforted Heleen with the promise that he would come and get her quickly when she was better. He was very concerned and kind to her. Heleen said nothing. She just looked terrified. When we got to the Wilhelmina Gasthuis, she wanted to run away. I tried to talk to her. "Now, don't do that, Heleen. We'll come to visit you this evening."

She silently allowed herself to be persuaded and went along to the ward.

The psychiatrist took a gloomy view of it. "When the psychosis is so far advanced that the patient no longer has any control over himself, as a rule the illness can't be arrested without compulsory hospitalization. I suspect that she will run away and I can't prevent that. That's why these cases are so difficult to treat."

"Is there nothing to be done in this case?" I asked. "At the moment she has no one who can look after her."

But his only answer was "Alas."

We left Heleen behind and promised to come as early as we could in the evening. But we didn't have to. She ran away within two hours. Raf went home with me. He said nothing. When I was telephoned by the Wilhelmina Gasthuis and told that Heleen wasn't there any more, Raf went to their house.

That same evening I had a phone call from one of the women from the commune where

Heleen had lived. She told me that Heleen had bought a train ticket to Maastricht and now had arrived at their place. "But we can't have her here in this state," she said.

"I understand that," I answered. "But I've been occupied for so long with Heleen that now I'm going to bow out. You probably know her mother. Now she's got to take her on."

"I don't think that's fair," said the voice at the other end. "You've got involved with her, and Heleen doesn't want anything to do with her mother."

"I can't do anything more about it here," I said emphatically. "I have done what I could."

For a few days after Heleen's departure I heard nothing more from Raf. Then he came regularly again. He didn't say much, nor did I ask anything. It did seem to me that in the beginning he appeared to suffer very little in Heleen's absence. On the contrary, he seemed freed of a hard task.

He said that now he would concentrate on his band.

Gradually I got to hear more about the situation in Heleen's house. It seemed now that a few young people led by Harry had settled in. They made a lot of noise and played records at night. The neighbors had warned them that they would file a complaint.

After this latest news Raf came less and less often to see me. Probably there was no possibility to sleep in a full house where it was lively at night, and he had to catch up on his sleep during the day.

When he came again after a few weeks, he looked bad and, because of a lack of medicine, it was difficult for him to concentrate, which was evident in long pauses between his sentences. "Heleen's mother has rented out the house," he said. "Now I live somewhere with Harry and his girlfriend." And that was all he said. He gazed straight ahead dreamily.

"Where do you live with Harry and his girlfriend?" I asked.

"At one of their friends'. I've got a corner of the living room where I can sleep."

After two months Heleen's mother phoned me. "You should have kept those two people apart instead of encouraging it," she said angrily. "But you naturally thought that such a nice girl would be good for him."

I understood her and couldn't say much in my defence. She was terribly worried about her daughter, who was roaming around Holland sick and neglected without anyone being able to detain her and persuade her to go into a hospital.

Later I heard that Heleen had made a suicide attempt and with a sectioning order was admitted to the institution where she had been cared for before.

Chapter 10   Bows and Bells

After three months Raf came back home to live. Harry had rented a room somewhere else and Raf didn't want to stay by himself with Harry's friend.

I expected that a more regular life in a warm house with his own room and a shower would do him good. In the beginning he obviously enjoyed all this luxury. He didn't hear much from Harry any more. Now and then in the youth club, where Raf still went regularly, people could play musical instruments. Raf smiled and said that Harry would get up on the stage with a harmonica and couldn't be got off it again for the whole evening.

When I asked him how it was going with Heleen, he didn't answer and looked straight ahead pensively.

Then there was a phone call. The voice on the other end was so soft that I could only understand the name "Raf". I called him. It proved to be Heleen on the telephone. Raf walked up and down nervously with the receiver at his ear. He kept saying very tensely, "Don't do it. I'm coming. I'm coming. I'm coming over. You must stay there. Heleen, you must stay put. I'm really coming over."

When he had hung up the telephone he burst out crying. "Heleen was talking such nonsense and was so pathetic," he said. "I can't help her when she's in this state, can I? I can't ask her to come back, can I? But she does want to come back and I feel so sorry for her. What can I do?"

I phoned the psychiatric institution where Heleen was being cared for and spoke with the head nurse. He knew who I was from the first words, for Heleen had often talked about Raf.

"She can't have any visitors yet," he said. "Certainly not Raf. Heleen was admitted here in a seriously sick condition and must still rest for a long time."

I had the impression that Raf felt relieved that for the time being he couldn't go to her. For a long time after that we heard nothing more from her.

Raf was just as lonely as before he had met Heleen and was only now realising that he missed her. Harry had also broken off contact since he had gone to live in his own flat with his girlfriend.

I had very often noticed that Raf considered admittance in an institution when he felt very lonely and not because he had any hopes for a cure. He wanted to be among people who he felt would understand him. Now he began to talk about it again.

"Yesterday I looked up a fellow in Santpoort," he said. "Maasland Section. I intend to get in there, too."

He had heard from friends the way to go about that and went to the Area Health Authority to discuss it with the psychiatrist, who already knew him well. He agreed with him and would get in touch with Maasland.

The Area Health Authority polyclinic was

also a social centre. When Raf felt bored he sometimes went there to see whether he could find old friends. In the morning there was a separate mental hygiene service where medicines could be collected and where consultations could be had without an appointment.

After the conversation about Maasland, Raf waited stoically for an answer and sat for almost the whole day in the same corner of the living room staring straight ahead.

Only with tasty food could I occasionally please him. Sometimes he also wanted to listen to records of Bach or Mozart in the evening. Now he couldn't stand any other music. He found it either too changeable in mood, which excited him, or it made him sad. In those days I was happy if a smile sometimes appeared on his face.

Finally word came that he could be placed. For the first time I felt apprehensive about it, especially because Maasland was a similar institution to Buiten Oord. When Raf had been admitted there eight years before, the age range varied from 15 to 21 years. I had seen what could happen within a few years: how the insidious decline could not be prevented. I was afraid that in Maasland, where the age limit was from about 22 to 35 years, this would be the case to an even greater degree.

Furthermore, my first visit didn't allay my fears.

Maasland was a building with three sections. On the ground floor was the department for new patients who were seriously ill. On the first floor improved patients were treated, and the top floor was for the patients to be discharged. On my arrival the outer door was opened with a key. I came into a grimy, dark hallway where tables, a couple of chairs, and a few benches stood. The people on the ground floor seemed to be so disturbed that there was no point in trying to talk to them. The nurse who had opened the door must have been in a great hurry, because she had immediately gone away with quick steps without introducing herself. After a few minutes I saw Raf, who came shuffling along. I noticed at once that he had gone downhill in the two weeks since I had last seen him. He chuckled when he came up to me, and all he said was, "I'm going to take a shower," and was off again.

In all possible places people lay sleeping. A boy was constantly hitting his head against the wall without anybody doing anything about it.

A man of about 35 kept going through the hallway as though he were a steam train. He hissed like an escape valve, louder and louder. That lasted for the whole hour without anyone paying any attention to him. A third boy was mooing like a cow.

Raf came from taking his shower and got dressed. He went to sit by me without saying anything and chuckled occasionally. "I'm going to take a shower," was the only thing that he said for the next half hour, and he disappeared for the second time.

I had had experience with all sorts of institutions, but I had never before seen so many

144

seriously disturbed people together. I took comfort in the thought that this section was meant only for short observation and that afterwards a treatment would begin.

After this first visit I went to see my psychiatrist again. I told him what I had seen and that Raf had spent the whole afternoon in the shower.

"I've heard that no medicines at all are given in this section," said the psychiatrist. "And these surroundings can't stimulate Raf to take part in activities, either. On the contrary, I think that so many disturbed people all together with whom he can hold absolutely no conversations make him extra anxious. You said that Raf also used to take a lot of showers when he didn't feel at ease. Now he probably has still more need to ward off his anxiety through compulsive washing. There are many indications that some patients try in this way to wash themselves clean of their anxiety-laden guilt feelings."

On my next visit I still wanted to meet the staff, but again there was nobody to be seen. Finally it turned out that the entire nursing staff were chatting in an office.

Raf went back and forth through the hallway with one hand raised limply, spoke incoherent words that I couldn't make out, and paid little attention to me. When he came past me he always said something to me as though he was conscious that he couldn't entirely ignore me. Then he would say, "You're here, are you?" and then walk on. The second time he said, more to himself than to me, "That's her, she's..." That showed me that he was occupied with thoughts connected with me.

When he came around again, I asked, "Why don't you come and sit down for a bit, Raf? I've come a long way to see you." That last remark got to him. He came and sat beside me.

I asked him where the patients lived and he looked at me blankly at first, but when I asked it again with emphasis he was a bit more lucid.

"Here in the hallway," he said.

I had seen that there were another couple of untidy little rooms: stuffy, little and dirty, with a few tables and chairs and unmade beds on which there were dirty sheets and blankets. I was never able to discover a dining room. The staff kept themselves so aloof that I had no opportunity to ask questions. If I did manage it, I was constantly directed to the psychiatrist. But in the six months that Raf had been admitted to Maasland I was never able to get to speak to a psychiatrist.

Quite soon Raf was allowed to go home for the weekend. That caused still more problems and there were moments when I panicked, like the time that he suddenly kicked a little table against the gas heater. The glass top shattered all over the room and Raf looked on triumphantly. Then he started laughing loudly.

Then he suddenly became angry and had an argument with someone in himself. I had only rarely seen him so angry. He was talking about "dirty trick" and "if you so much as dare". I could do nothing and phoned the institution to say that

Raf's behavior at the weekends was impossible to put up with. But the nursing staff said that when he was at home I must take responsibility and that I must get in touch with the psychiatrist if I wanted to make a complaint.

In all these months Raf's situation only got worse. Nothing changed in the clinic, either. Every time I went there I saw the man who thought he was a train still going hissing through the hallway like a steam locomotive; and the man who thought he was a cow was still mooing.

The following weekend Raf came home with coloured bows on his coat and bells around his neck.

"Did the staff let you go out like that?" I asked.

He simply said, "Yes."

When he took off his coat, he carefully pinned all the bows on his sweater and put the bells around his neck. He had hardly any contact with the outside world any more. His foolish laugh made him unrecognizable to me.

Sometimes he stayed away on weekends. Then I went to visit him anyway, although I wondered whether he had trouble there. When he was feeling a bit better he said that there was a lot of quarrelling among the patients and that he would rather leave. I didn't know what to say about that. It seemed to me unthinkable to have Raf at home in this state. He had chosen Maasland and I still expected one or another treatment eventually.

But a week after that he came home with loads of baggage. When I asked him about all the stuff he had with him, he reacted with such a furious look that I just let it drop.

What he unpacked startled me. A few pairs of shoes and boots, a good ten pairs of trousers and sweaters, and about twenty-five gramophone records.

"Raf, who does all this belong to?" I asked in amazement. But he looked at me so menacingly that I didn't say anything else and phoned the institution.

"The patients themselves must deal with these things," I was told by the management. "If they give things away or let them be taken away from them that is their own responsibility."

Later Raf only said, "My guitar is gone." Then I understood more. "I'm not going back again, either. I was nearly murdered last week."

I thought that his guitar going missing caused this nervous reaction, and I asked what exactly had happened.

"I was sitting on the toilet and hadn't locked the door," he said. "Suddenly a guy jumped me, and he began to scratch me and bite me, and he tried to strangle me."

I took the story for just that and didn't believe that this could be possible in an institution.

In the evening after the meal Raf was somewhat calmer. He sat in his pyjamas at the fireside. His pyjama top was open and I was deeply shocked by what I saw. His body was black and blue.

"What is the meaning of this?" I asked him. "Just take your top off for a minute."

The bites he had mentioned were clearly visible, and at his throat there were bruises that I hadn't seen before because he had been wearing a scarf.

Raf put his pyjama top back on and said, "I told you that I was nearly strangled."

He sat resignedly at the fireside. I wondered what was going to become of him. Suddenly that strength came back to me again that I had often felt when everything was going wrong. I said, "Raf, if you don't want to go back, then just stay at home. We'll see how it goes."

He looked at me and didn't answer, but I noticed in the way he changed position that a tension had fallen away from him.

He stayed at home but didn't know what to do with his time. He loafed about forlornly in the streets and didn't have any contact with anyone any more. Only the youth club in the city still offered him possibilities. Sometimes it seemed as if he spent day and night there. I let everything take its course. There was no longer any order in his life. He ran his days together. Sometimes I had the feeling that he almost didn't exist, so aloof, dreamy, and quiet he was.

I asked him once what he had done in the youth club. "I don't know – slept I think," he answered.

In the meantime Heleen had apparently turned up in the club, having run away from the institution. Raf had brought her home with him. She had put on a lot of weight and her pupils were so small that it seemed as though she wasn't looking with the same eyes that used to be so expressive. Two long snot candles ran down her nose into her mouth. She spoke with a thick tongue. It was winter and she wasn't wearing a coat. I gave her a heavy jacket and tried to explain to her that she would have to go back, but I got the feeling that she didn't understand me. Raf asked me for a handkerchief for her and there was something touching about the way he wiped her nose.

I knew that he had taken on a task that would be too hard for him. He tried as well as he could to take care of her. I think that he saw that as his duty, and at the same time he was happy to have something to do.

Heleen stayed with Raf for a couple of days. I didn't see her again after that. I think she slept all day.

But in spite of their limited possibilities for conversation, they still managed to plan to go together to the commune where Heleen had originally come from and had always wanted to go back to and had talked about with so much affection.

They took some possessions with them for their trip with the aim of staying longer.

But within a few days Raf came back. The commune had not given him permission to stay there longer. Heleen had already caused them enough problems.

I had the impression that Raf was satisfied with this outcome. He also said that they had discovered when they got to the commune that they had left all their baggage on the train. They hadn't enquired about it either, although there were valuable things in it. Nor did Raf want me to meddle in it.

"Oh, never mind, they were just material things," he said.

When he phoned Heleen again after a week, he learned that she was back in the hospital. Raf now thought once more about a new stay in hospital for himself, but this time I advised him against it. As long as he was looking at alternative institutions with a view to being admitted, I saw only disaster ahead. Up until now he had always been sicker when he came back out.

I gave him some more medicine in his food and tried to stimulate him by letting him paint the kitchen. He would get money for that to buy a new guitar. He thought that it was a good idea, set to work now and then, but was ashamed of his inability to do it. His isolation continued. After a month he came up with another scheme. He wanted to go to Israel again and work on a kibbutz there. The fresh air would do him good, he said, and he really ought to begin to think about his future.

I had become so discouraged that I could do nothing but wait and see resignedly how things would develop. Anyway, there seemed no other possible alternative.

Raf himself saw to his travel documents. He acted more lively and active again because of his new plan.

It turned out that the "Agency" that arranged the placement in kibbutzim had not given him permission because of his bad mental condition. They phoned me about it and advised me against letting Raf undertake this trip. The GP also thought it was a dubious business. But Raf went anyway. He would arrange to find a job, he said.

An acquaintance of mine even gave him a letter to take with him for a psychiatrist friend, in case he should get into difficulties. I had mixed feelings. Now that he was persevering so, I felt that I could believe in miracles again after all. I had a little hope that Raf might really stick it out for a while in Israel. Maybe he would even get better or at the very worst he would be hospitalized. Maybe there were psychiatrists there who could help him.

But when Raf arrived in Jerusalem it proved to be too crowded and too hot for him. He couldn't cope with all these stimuli and got so upset that he had the greatest trouble to keep going. After a few days he took the plane back.

In Switzerland he had to change planes, and while he was waiting he went somewhere around the airport to lie in the grass. He was very confused and talked to himself a lot, as I later heard from the Swiss authorities.

The Israeli stewardess, who had also been concerned about Raf on the plane, said that he mustn't lie there. Then he went to sit on a bench, for the plane wouldn't be leaving for more than an hour. Policemen wanted to take him away because they probably thought that they were faced with a drug addict. Raf gave them his passport to show that everything was all right. He said that he couldn't go with them because he was waiting for his plane to Amsterdam.

The policemen tried to take him anyway. Raf began to resist, was handcuffed, run in, and thrown into a cell. The whole night there he yanked at his handcuffs and cried, first out of fear of being alone and finally because his wrists were badly hurt. They let him scream and cry and didn't find it necessary to get a doctor. The police knew perfectly well what had to be done. Raf was bandaged the next day. He had 500 guilders with him. The money was taken from him and he got 25 guilders to take back home with him. At home he felt very low for a long time. What had happened kept swirling through his head. He kept asking me why they had treated him like that.

My GP wrote a letter to the Dutch embassy in Zürich in which he informed them that Raf must not be prosecuted because he was mentally disturbed. We got a letter back with an official penalty writ. So many extra legal expenses had been incurred that there were only 200 guilders left over. Raf would get them back only if he did not come in contact with the law for a year.

I indignantly phoned the embassy and said that a boy who shouldn't have been charged by the police in the first place should not have any conditions on his discharge.

However, some back-and-forth chitchat continued until at length I'd had enough of it.

Chapter 11 Apollo

In one of Raf's more lucid periods in which the mist around him lifted and he took an interest in friends and family, I told him that one of his friends was at university, another would soon become a father, and a third was already a doctor.

His eyes filled with tears and it seemed that a moment of lucidity caused even greater pain than his dim existence. What he had heard had taken him so much by surprise that he again looked dazed and quickly ducked back into his safer world, where the contours were fainter and he didn't have to feel so acutely how his life had gone wrong. But yet there were still days when he hoped once more to be able to do everything that he had planned to do.

Sometimes when we were talking together he idealized me in a way that struck me as uncomfortable. I was the best, the most interesting, most beautiful, and most sensible mother. I often had the feeling that that was his way of making it clear to me that he was devoted to me and that I mustn't abandon him. Later it would come out how deeply he was bound to me.

But there were also other moments in which his behaviour took terrifying forms. One night he knocked on my bedroom door, which I always kept locked. "Mum," he called, "where can I buy a knife sharpener?"

"Go to sleep," I called back. "It's the middle of the night. The shops aren't open until tomorrow morning."

I hoped that he would forget all about it. But when I got up that morning Raf had apparently already been out. He had not only bought a knife sharpener but also a big butcher knife that he was busy sharpening.

I looked, said nothing, and wondered if I was now really afraid. But to my amazement that seemed not to be the case.

When we were having breakfast Raf ate with his big knife. Also at lunch and at dinner he had it lying next to him. I considered what I ought to do and tucked it away. After that, each time I tried to put it somewhere harder to find, so that he would have to go to more and more trouble to find it.

Sometimes he asked, "Where's my knife?"

That went on for a couple of weeks until he gradually began to lose interest in it and asked about it less and less. Finally he ate again with his ordinary cutlery.

My psychiatrist thought that I had dealt with it well by not showing any fear. "In the end we don't know what plans Raf is really going around with," he said. "Probably there were voices that had given him orders. Because you handled it calmly, he was not compelled to carry out his order immediately, and he has therefore perhaps gradually come back to reality."

Raf told me that sometimes he slept in youth hostels.

"Why do you do that?" I asked. "It costs money, doesn't it, and you have a house, don't you?"

But he didn't answer. I had the impression that he was increasingly afraid to sleep alone in his room, but didn't always want to let it show. Perhaps he also had a need to be with other people. He stayed away when it suited him, and because I noticed that he kept coming back unharmed, I gradually stopped worrying about it, even when I heard nothing from him for weeks. All I knew was that there was a good chance that he would come home completely confused and sometimes strangely rigged out. It did make me anxious when I heard that he was sleeping in the Vondel Park, because in those days it was a very violent place.

One morning I noticed that he was very emotional. His walls were covered with writing with unclear sentences in which, taking a quick glance at it, I could recognise words.

"Another world...where sun...dead...everywhere...really is..." It went on: "Is not...Isn't it?...is it?...or not?...or totally?...it is really...it is...is it?...it's not...or is it?...or not?..."

The room was in great disorder and I saw that Raf had been crying. Finally I discovered his new guitar among the mess. He had kicked it to pieces.

"Why did you do that?" I asked.

He began to cry again and said that he didn't know. "I saw it lying broken on the floor this morning," he said.

He told me that he kept hearing loud voices that frightened him. Also, with increasing frequency things happened that he couldn't remember.

Suddenly I learned that Raf had requested admittance to Eden Oord (another institution in Santpoort) and that he would leave a week later. I was no longer astonished by it; I was just afraid of the difficulties that would arise again.

In the meantime the dark days before Christmas were upon us. They were a difficult time for Raf, in which as a rule he became depressed. On New Year's Eve he came home for two days. He looked calm. There was an easy-going smile on his face. He sat down and waited for me to sit down.

"Something strange has happened," he said. "I've met an apparition of you."

I asked him if he could tell something about it and he began to talk with great concentration.

"I was walking with you on the beach," he said. "The weather was beautiful. You were, too. We walked for a long time. It got quiet and a bit dark. You stopped and asked me to kiss you passionately. When I did that, I gradually went completely inside your belly. There were also two girls there, Hooloofoo and Dilifie, really sweet girls. We were born again. You told us that we had come from another world, a world of a long time ago, and that it would be difficult for us to live here in this world. We came from Apollo, you said. You told us to try it here. I had to kiss you again and when I next looked at you, you had turned into sand. You were a pillar of sand. You were just like Lot's wife. Suddenly Jonah's whale swallowed us up. Now, fortunately, all three of us are back in this time. The girls Hooloofoo and Dilifie are staying in the Apollo Hotel. I can't leave them alone on New Year's Eve, so I'm going to stay there too. Life here is very strange for them, so I have to help them. They aren't terribly out-going girls. They're quite mild-mannered."

He had told the story in a relaxed way, looked at his watch, put his boots and coat on, and left. When he said good-bye he added, "I'll come and see you around twelve to wish you a Happy New Year."

After a while I rang the Apollo Hotel and it appeared that Raf had, in fact, arrived there. The reception had found it quite strange but had seen no reason to refuse him. He had paid in advance.

We had been invited with the whole family to go to the house of some friends this New Year's Eve. A few minutes before midnight Raf did indeed ring the doorbell. We were standing all ready with a glass of champagne. He came in with the bulbous room key from the Apollo Hotel in his hand.

"I can only stay a minute," he said. "I promised to come right back. The girls feel uncomfortably alone here."

He stayed for 15 minutes and left after he had given us all his best wishes.

The next morning he came home. I noticed that his mood had definitely taken a downturn. He now looked disturbed. He looked nervously around and I saw that he was looking for something.

Later it turned out that he was looking for two little woollen crocheted dolls, each one a bit larger than a hand. I had once crocheted the dolls for the children. For Sabina a black girl with a bun, and for Raf a blonde girl with hair hanging loose. They had always hung on the wall in their rooms as mascots.

When Raf came into the living room again he had a bulge under his shirt. I asked him what it was. He looked irritated and said, "Oh, nothing."

Since he had not completely closed his shirt, I saw later that the two crocheted dolls hung against his abdomen on a string, held in place by his trouser belt. He carried those dolls with him for years. They evidently meant a lot to him, for he didn't forget them even in his most difficult period.

The very same day he went back to Eden Oord, sad and lonely, with the dolls under his shirt against his stomach.

My psychiatrist spoke with me in some detail about Raf's story. He found it a classic example of a hallucinatory condition. "It is curious that Raf, who is always so closed up, now for the first time exposed his feelings. During the whole story he was in a blissful dream world. Can you figure out how he came up with these fanciful names?" he asked.

"When the children were small I taught them a secret language," I said. "Every syllable was lengthened with loofoo, lafa, lofo, lefe, or lifi. So "papa" became *palafapalafa*, "mother" became *molofothelefer*, and the word "reopen" would be *relefeolofopelefen*. My children quickly became

159

very skilful in this language and often spoke it. 'Hooloofoo' must be Heleen in this case, although it doesn't entirely tally with our language. But then, it seems to me unlikely that Raf would still remember the details. What 'Dilifi' means I don't know."

"What Raf says in his dream is naturally obvious to you, too. In his vision he had sexual relations with you. He had two children from that. One of them is thus his girlfriend. Dilifie is in my opinion Delphi, the Greek oracle where the god Apollo was worshiped. Raf has had, as you said, a classical education. He knows what Delphi means, namely 'womb'. Also it's no coincidence that he chose the Apollo Hotel to stay in with the two daughters that he sired with his mother, that is, with you. Apollo is also the god of music and poetry. Raf had great respect for you in his dream. You warned him that it would be difficult for the three of them in this world. So you understood him. What other meanings he may have attached to Apollo are not entirely clear; about that only Raf himself would be able to enlighten us. Perhaps it also has something to do with the time when he was well, when he was still at the Gymnasium. When he kissed you for the second time, you changed into a pillar of sand.

"That is obviously connected with the Bible story of Lot's wife, who turned into a rigid pillar of salt when she looked back at the cities of Sodom and Gomorrah, which were infested with homosexuality and then were engulfed by fire and brimstone. Raf made a pillar of sand from that, which corresponds with the stone figure that resembles a woman on the shore of the Dead Sea and which is called 'Lot's Wife'. We know that Lot himself was seduced by his daughters so as not to let his family line die out. The incest motif clearly plays a part here again.

"The punishment for this also follows at once. Jonah's whale swallows up Raf and the daughters, whom he created with his mother, including Hooloofoo, who in any case also represents his girlfriend. In the Bible Jonah is punished in that way because he has resisted the commandments of God. Clearly the guilt feelings that Raf has about his erotic desires in regard to you are involved here. Raf cannot leave the two girls alone in the Apollo Hotel and he goes to them. It is striking that he says how mild-mannered they are.

"He has also always done his best to make his mildness prevail. That also explains his blissful feeling. Through the two girls that he has made himself, he can free himself from his anxiety and from his aggression. He slept that night with his own, nonexistent, daughter and girlfriend who were born from incest. The next day he comes back. He carries the two dolls, which naturally must represent the two girls, under his shirt on his abdomen, perhaps meaning an identification of Raf with the mother figure. In that way the need to give birth to himself could be manifested. That happens a lot with schizophrenics. They often split up the feminine and masculine sides in themselves."

When I visited Raf a week later with Hans, he walked past us. He glanced at us as though he had already seen us once before. We waited a moment, but it was clear that he wanted no approach at all. We therefore decided to go away and to get in touch afterwards with the psychiatrist in charge, a young woman who saw us on our next visit. She was an intern training in Eden Oord and had seen Raf only a few times.

She could tell us nothing about him.

Raf himself now recognised us, came to us for a moment, mumbled a couple of incomprehensible words, made a warding-off gesture with his hand as though he had had enough of it, and disappeared again.

Afterwards we heard nothing more from him for a while. We decided not to go to see him as long as he was still in this psychotic condition. When I rang up the clinic and asked how he was, I felt strongly that there was a reluctance to divulge information.

But after about a month I was rung up by a social worker. He was keen for a confrontation with Raf and me, and he said that with a cheerful voice as though something pleasant was going to happen.

He received me in a lovely sunny room. Raf was already sitting there. "How do you like it that your mother is here?" asked the social worker.

Raf burst out into uncontrollable laughter.

"Why must you laugh like that?" asked the social worker.

"You are a silly blonde," answered Raf.

I had never before seen him so uncooperative.

"Is that why you laugh like that?" asked the social worker with a serious expression.

As an answer Raf laughed still louder.

Years before, when his illness was not yet apparent, he had already had a gift for seeing through people. Now he must also have had the feeling that the pompous manner of his social worker was unnecessary.

"Your son is in a good mood," said the social worker brightly.

"I see that," was my answer.

Thereupon he turned again to Raf and asked, "Won't you talk to your mother?"

Raf took his scarf, on which were printed little coloured balls, from his neck and said, "Bang, Mum, look out, bang! All the little balloons on this scarf say 'bang'. Duck, here comes another one, look out! Bang. Bang. Bang. Ouch, duck!"

I understood very well that Raf was expressing aggression toward me, but I had the still stronger feeling that he found the whole business a farce and he was expressing this by his manner.

"Raf evidently has something against you," observed the social worker.

"When a son is as sick as Raf is, of course he must have had the feeling that I had abandoned him over the years. I am of course a mother, but still just an ordinary person. I think that I've fallen short of the images that he must have had of me in his hallucinatory states. Is that by any chance what you mean?"

But he didn't answer that and turned again to Raf. "Why don't you want to talk to your mother?"

Raf kept laughing and repeated, "Bang. Bang. Bang. Nice scarf, eh?"

Now I began to get angry about this ridiculous situation. "Will you listen to *me* for a moment?" I said to the social worker. "Raf has now been sick for almost eleven years. In that time he has been in all kinds of unreal situations. Nothing surprises me any more. But now I do want to know why you have had me come here. I understand that it's your job and you have to fill up your time. You're earning money from this pointless hour. I hope that you know that you're barking up the wrong tree. I don't want to have any more to do with this. My experience with Raf's illness has gradually become too extensive for that. What you think you have discovered, among other things that Raf has aggressive feelings toward me, is obvious to me. There are so many young people who are aggressive toward their parents, but they are not all mentally disturbed by it. If you give Raf medicine for a week so that he is somewhat more approachable again, you can phone me again."

I said good-bye and left.

I felt that I was expected to take part in every experiment the therapists happened to think up. But I was tired with all the experimenting. I had already had so much experience of it that I couldn't believe in it any more.

As unexpectedly as Raf had got himself admitted to the institution, he came back with all his baggage. He had been in Eden Oord for four months in all. He gave no explanation but just kept laughing a lot. In this situation there was no talking to him, so I just waited to see what would happen.

I could no longer go on living with Raf. I could not resign myself to the fact that I couldn't lead my own life in my own house and that this would have to go on like this, without hope.

Chapter 12   Autism

That winter Raf lay for days on end in front of the hearth without any contact with anyone at all. He was always falling asleep while he was smoking and there were big holes in the rug.

When I would talk about it with my psychiatrist he would say that he couldn't help me.

It had been a long time since I had invited people over. I didn't dare do it any more. Raf's behaviour seemed to be too painful for them. But I also noticed that my need to talk about Raf's illness with other people increased, for because of their discomfort with the situation I was in danger of getting more and more isolated.

The maximum amount of medicine that I now dared to give Raf appeared to be just enough to keep his most dangerous behaviour somewhat in check. His psychiatrist said that the medicines that he now needed would have to be sorted out in a clinic.

Latterly I was staying as long as possible at my work. When I came home either Raf lay asleep or he was out. I had already very often thought that if anything should ever happen to him, it would be a long time before I found out about it. Mostly he stayed away for a short time, but it also happened that he didn't come home for days, or even weeks. For that reason I used to hide little notes in his pockets with our address on them. He now often forgot his house key, too. By this time I had got used to sleeping with earplugs so as not to be constantly confronted by his nocturnal restlessness. For that reason I couldn't hear the bell if he came home in the middle of the night.

Sometimes he threw pebbles against the window, because that did wake me up. But there were a couple of times when he didn't have enough energy to throw pebbles and fell asleep in the outer hallway. That even happened twice in the winter. I then cut out a big key from red paper and stuck it on the wall of the hallway so that he couldn't miss it when he was leaving our house. Even that didn't help.

One morning, after Raf had been roaming around somewhere for a couple of days, Hans phoned from The Hague. Raf had rung his doorbell in the middle of the night, and when it wasn't opened fast enough he had thrown a stone through the window. Hans had heard nothing, for his bedroom was at the back of the top floor. But new neighbours, who didn't know Raf and thought that it was a burglar, had called the police.

Another time when he was in The Hague, Raf had rung up his father in the middle of the night again and asked whether he could come and get him.

"What's *got* into you?" Hans had answered. "You *got* me up."

"Two thousand years ago you also forsook me," Raf had replied.

He continued to identify with the Christ figure, who while on the cross had also wondered whether God had forsaken him. With Raf I had the feeling that, as far as his attitude toward his father was concerned, he compared himself with Christ. Hans suffered acutely from that.

Hans understood how desperate the situation was for me and tried to help me sometimes by keeping Raf in The Hague for a while when possible. But he also had two growing children at home, so it was not without problems.

My feelings of guilt and sympathy toward Raf were greater as it became clearer to me that I wanted to be free of him. I considered that Raf would just have to learn to live by himself if no other possibility could be found. I was now increasingly occupied with these thoughts.

Raf would never be in a state to find a house by himself, and no landlord would take him on as a tenant. But I found out that there was a section of the Social Services for those seeking accommodation who were socially inadequate.

"What would you think about having a place of your own?" I asked Raf. But just as I had expected, he didn't react. He only looked at me with big anxious eyes and left the room.

I understood that he was afraid to live alone, and I let the plan drop for a while. However, there were circumstances that made the situation acute again. Once during lunchtime, as we were eating, I could barely get Raf out of the conversation that he was having with himself. He just moved his mouth and was inaudible. I had already spoken to him twice, but he kept saying "Shh" and waving his hand as a sign that I mustn't interrupt him. After a while I tried it again.

He slowly raised his head. I saw that he

was looking at me in a strange way. There was something ominous in his look. He gave me the impression that he was dreaming with his eyes open. He put his hands flat on the table, slowly stood up, and suddenly gave me such a powerful shove that I was thrown against the corner of the kitchen counter. Nothing like that had ever happened before. I was taken by surprise and screamed. This probably encouraged him. He began to hit me, and every time I tried to take a step he would knock me against the counter. Through my pain I felt that something must happen to stop him.

My anger began to overcome my fear. Suddenly I yelled very loudly: "Are you completely out of your bloody mind? Cut it out! Do you hear?"

This reaction brought him back to his senses a bit. He stopped, and in his confusion I managed to get away.

My neighbour, who had heard the uproar, was standing in the hallway. I ran into her flat and asked her to shut the door. I now felt a severe pain in my back and bruising was visible. But I realised that, now that the illness had taken this turn, I would no longer feel safe around Raf. But before I could think any further he knocked on the door.

"Will you please listen to me?" he asked imploringly. "Mum, please believe me. It wasn't you. I didn't hit you. It really wasn't you," he called through the door.

I opened the door. "I would never hit you," he continued. "You know that I would never do that, don't you?"

He looked so miserable that I immediately went upstairs with him again. Now he was crying. I believed him and understood that he too realized that he was now capable of acts that he had to carry out against his will.

"Something will indeed have to happen now to avoid serious consequences," my psychiatrist said. "Raf doesn't know what to do with his aggression towards you. He suffers from his guilt feelings. He is dependent on you, would like to be nice to you, but yet feels abandoned by you. It must have been a great shock for him that you didn't want to have him with you any more and that you tried to find a house for him. His conscience says that he must be nice to you, but his vindictiveness, which is revealed in aggression, compels him to do the opposite."

I discussed the situation with a family member who was familiar with council housing. I told him that, although I doubted whether Raf would ever have the courage to live in his own house, there was no other solution except to try it. I got in touch with the relevant department and was requested to write a letter about the urgency of Raf's case. I received an answer quickly. They found my situation obviously a priority case.

Within three months Raf got word that he had to come and talk. But at that moment he couldn't reply because he was too mixed up and too ill. So I went there myself and asked if they could postpone the thing for a little while.

That was done, but the housing that had

been earmarked for Raf couldn't be reserved for him. However, they did promise me that a new offer would come along shortly.

Now I tried to help Raf in every possible way. I bought plates and cups for the new house, but it didn't do any good. Only when I said that, all the same, it would be nice for him if his friend Eddy would come and live with him after his discharge from the institution, did Raf take more interest in the project. Although he rarely heard anything from Eddy, he continued to believe in his return to normal society. It appeared to me that he needed this trust to keep going himself.

From Eddy's mother, whom I sometimes phoned, I heard that she was at the end of her tether with him. He made life for her and his father unbearable, kept running away from the institution, hit his mother, made a mess of the house, and broke up the furniture. But whatever his parents did, they could never get an order for compulsory admittance to hospital. Eddy got more and more ill. With each contact with the Area Health Authority his parents heard the same thing: "The patient must have inflicted on himself or others a dangerous injury. Otherwise it is not possible for the Area Health Authority to intervene or submit an application for a sectioning order."

When Raf had improved somewhat, he himself rang up the Social Services department for housing-seekers. He stuttered during the conversation. He had been doing this for a little while and just when he was somewhat less confused than usual. I had the impression that in his more lucid moments he felt his lack of skill in things that had earlier come easily for him. He went on with the conversation, didn't let himself get discouraged by the fact that he had trouble finishing his sentences, and he spoke very realistically. He made an appointment with a social worker who would help him with renting a house.

When she came to us to talk to him, Raf seemed to get along well with her.

Now there was again available housing that he could qualify for, close to me in our neighbourhood, because the Social Services thought it better for Raf not to feel too lonely and to be able to visit me easily.

The landlord was happy to take Raf on as a tenant if Social Services would stand surety for the rent, and it was agreed that the rent would be paid directly by the Services to the landlord and then deducted from Raf's benefit payment.

Hans and I furnished the house for Raf. He, however, put off living in it from day to day, until he finally said, sadly, that he would try it after all.

The house had two main rooms and a little room between them. In each room we put a bed, because we knew that Raf would often bring guests home. As the one valuable object, he brought along an amplifier that he had just bought and on which there were all kinds of knobs and buttons.

Because he found it difficult to stay alone at night, he soon invited a fellow from the youth club to stay with him. The next day he had breakfast with him. The fellow took a shower first and then

Raf. When he came out of it the guy had disappeared with the amplifier.

I had already warned Raf repeatedly that he couldn't trust everyone, but he had just shaken his head and said, "It's not nice to think badly of people."

In spite of his experience he continued to believe in people. It sometimes seemed as though he needed that belief in order not to be completely alone in his sorry existence. But because of that he was repeatedly abused. Within a week he came home again.

"I can't keep on living there," he said. "My neighbour is a murderer. I've seen a trail of blood on the stairs!" I knew that on the first three steps a couple of small, red flecks of paint had been spilled. I remember that I thought at the time, "If only Raf doesn't get frightened about them."

I tried to accept his return as calmly as possible. It had by then become spring and I hoped that, as the days got longer, Raf would settle down a bit better in his own house.

His psychiatrist gave me new medicines that went with the kind that Raf already used, but substances were now added that should yield a better result for his autism. At first Raf reacted well to them, but in the end his suspicion grew and after two weeks he became anxious.

The psychiatrist advised me to be careful. "You must understand," he said, "that medicines have a considerable effect on the body. The patient may indeed suffer great anxiety if he doesn't know why he feels different."

Now, just as before, Raf crept up slyly behind me when I was working in the kitchen to see what I was doing with the food. Gradually I saw his behaviour change. Again for entire nights he didn't go to bed but played the guitar and sang along so loudly that I couldn't sleep. I decreased the amount of medication. But Raf still kept exhibiting decidedly paranoid behaviour.

He now also very often went out to eat. When he sometimes ate at home he looked searchingly at his plate and tasted his food very carefully. A new hallucination must have taken hold of him. During one of our meals he suddenly said, "They put poison in the food of a guy I know."

After that he ate every evening in a community centre and paid for it by washing dishes.

Now and then he slept in his own house, but it was always hard for him. I think that he did it only because he paid rent, and so he thought that he should put the house to some use.

I had resolved that, in any case, I would go on holiday and decided to install a new lock on the door to prevent finding on my return, as in all other years, the great disorder caused by the invasion of Raf's acquaintances. So he would have to get used to his own house. But this again proved to be a miscalculation. When I came back Hans picked me up at the airport and I saw at once that something was wrong.

"What's happened with Raf?" I asked

anxiously.

"Oh, nothing," he answered.

"What is it then?"

He tried to change the subject and I didn't manage to find out anything more. Near my house Raf was sitting on the steps of the city library. He looked sad, confused and neglected.

I felt a stab in my heart and instantly forgot my vacation. The guilt feelings and the hopelessness of the situation once again came at me undiminished. Hans told me that during my absence Raf had been badly confused and that for two weeks he had sat on the step of the library every day waiting for the tram that would bring me back. When this didn't happen, since he couldn't get into the house, he chiselled out around the locks of all the doors. It was only when I was about to go into my house that I noticed what had happened.

The wood was carefully cut away and the doors, which were lacking a square piece around the lock, stood open. The locks were attached to the doorjambs with the wood still there. Raf had done that to three doors. It looked sinister and it clearly reflected how aggressive and hopeless he must have felt.

When I asked him why he had done that, he only said, "I couldn't get in." He looked dreamily straight ahead, as though he had nothing to do with all this.

I had got rid of the misery for a while and now I felt panic rise in me. I wanted to go away, to bear no more responsibility, to have no more guilt feelings. I wanted to be somewhere else. An uncontrollable weariness overcame me and I just wanted to sleep. It had now been plainly demonstrated that Raf couldn't manage for a moment without me. I had expected that something would surely change now that he had a new house, but in this way he had made it clear to me that I should expect nothing from him. How would he ever cope with life by himself? How could *I* have a life of my own? These thoughts kept turning around in my mind.

When I told my brother about the reception at home, he screwed steel plates on the outside door to give me a feeling of safety.

When I looked at Raf's sad face and saw that joyless life in him, I again felt inclined to devote myself to him. At the same time I felt still more strongly that I wouldn't be able to keep that up in the long run. Much greater difficulties and dangers would not fail to materialize.

In the meantime Raf tried again to see if he could manage to live in his house, but something always went wrong. One time a fellow he had brought in didn't want to go away and said, "You have enough room and I don't have a house."

"But my friend Eddy is coming here to live," Raf had answered.

He then came to me and said that he didn't want to stay with that fellow. I had to call the police in to force him to leave.

After that another fellow came with four girls from France. He wanted to have them stay with Raf because it had become known that he had room. Raf had no peace and quiet in his house and repeatedly sought refuge with me. Every time I had to go to the greatest trouble to get the intruders out of his house and get the key back from them. It looked as though Raf sought these complications. I saw how he relaxed with me at home without all those problems around him, and again I fought with my guilt feelings.

Finally he said that he wouldn't go to his house again before his neighbour, the murderer, had left. "I don't feel like becoming his next victim."

So he was staying with me again for good, and I hoped for a miracle because I had nothing else to hope for. As a rule Raf was uncommunicative, but sometimes he had moods in which he kept talking non-stop and couldn't be silenced. One afternoon he suddenly said, "Mum, you mustn't *ever* leave me. You must always stay with me. You're the only one I've got."

I had a feeling of being strangled and felt myself become breathless. It was obvious. There were mothers who would see this as their duty. Why couldn't I summon up that feeling? But I felt that I couldn't make this concession.

"Raf," I said. "I think it's really sweet when a boy of seven says something like that, but a fellow of 27…that's not on. I won't always be here. Something could suddenly happen to me and you would have to go on regardless. That's also the reason that you've got a house. You'll have to learn to look after yourself. I've done it up until now, but you're too old now and I can't cope with it any more."

There was a long silence. Then Raf went off to his nursery, where he had been sleeping lately. That evening I asked him, as usual, to come and eat, but he didn't answer. He lay in his bed, curled up with his knees against his chin and his thumb in his mouth. It reminded me of Heleen. She had lain just like this, like a baby, on the bench at the A and E.

The next morning Raf didn't respond to my request to come and eat breakfast. When he didn't eat or drink all day, I rang Hans in The Hague.

He would come as fast as possible.

We both agreed that Raf had to be admitted again.

A friend of Hans' had become the director of a psychiatric institution near Rotterdam. Hans phoned him and explained the urgency of the case. The new director was willing to take Raf into his clinic, but before that the ordinary procedure had to be followed.

The next day there was no change in Raf's behaviour, although Hans did manage to get some food into his mouth and get him to drink something. If *I* gave him anything he remained motionless, as though I didn't exist.

Two days later we went to the Area Health Authority to arrange Raf's admittance. Through all the difficulties I had forgotten that Mrs. Raas, the psychiatrist in charge, might meet me. All of a sudden I was standing in front of her.

When I told her the latest development in Raf's illness, she reacted in her own sarcastic manner. As though she had spoken to me only yesterday, she said, "Yes, Mrs. Anstadt, here we are again with your little boy, because you haven't wanted to let him go. We can do nothing for you. There's no room."

"I've been in touch with the director of the Bertus Clinic," Hans put in. "He's prepared to admit Raf."

"So," said Mrs. Raas with an amiable smile, "that's fine. And is Raf also prepared for that?"

Hans still tried to make the seriousness of the situation clear to her, but she didn't react to that and wasn't willing to help us. We went back home without having achieved anything.

Through my work I had regular contact with a psychiatrist who was also in the management of the Area Health Authority. Although I often met him at meetings, I had never yet talked to him about Raf. But now I told him everything.

"I'll see what I can do for you," he said. "Just phone Mrs. Raas again tomorrow for a new appointment."

The next day she did behave somewhat less dismissively on the telephone. This time I went with my brother to the Area Health Authority. My fear of Mrs. Raas had become so great in all those years that I knew that I wouldn't be able to say a word to her myself. Even in my greatest desperation I had never yet heard anything friendly from her, and I wasn't the only one.

We came into a packed waiting room where patients were walking around restlessly and telling each other in a raucous tone of voice the most improbable stories. Others sat still, staring into space in a world of their own.

I didn't know this new building. The waiting room was too little for this large group of people. The old one, in which I had often sat with Raf, had been very big and all the noise could be absorbed by the space.

After an hour calm had returned. We were the only ones who were still waiting. After we had waited for more than two hours my brother became furious at this unseemly behaviour. He went to ring for all the authorities in the building. Finally Mrs. Raas came. She didn't find it necessary to apologize.

"Do you have something new?" she asked in a business-like tone.

My brother wanted to begin a conversation but he didn't get a chance. "You surely can't deal with this case like this?" he said.

"I don't know what else should happen with it. You must have permission from Raf for admittance."

And we went away for the second time without having achieved anything.

After a week there was still no change in Raf's condition. He ate only if Hans fed him, and he had to come from The Hague to do it.

At my wit's end, I rang up the psychiatrist from my work again. I got his wife, a social worker, on the phone. I don't know how long I talked to her. I poured out everything that had become too much for me. I cried and asked her if *she* knew any way out.

"Raf's father lives in The Hague," I said. "Something really has to happen. Raf surely can't starve to death? His father now comes to Amsterdam every day to feed him, and there's no noticeable change at all in his condition."

She promised me to talk about it with her husband and to do everything that lay in her power to help.

The following day I was phoned by Dr. van Thuyl of the Area Health Authority. He would come to visit us to talk to Raf.

When he went into Raf's room the next day, Raf suddenly woke up. "Will you get out of my room?" he said. "You have no business here."

"I came to talk to you," the doctor began. "We think it would be better if you had yourself admitted to a hospital for a little while."

"I have nothing to do with you, and I'm not having myself admitted," Raf answered.

The psychiatrist came slowly and pensively into the living room. He made a calm impression, which dispelled my fear that again nothing would happen.

By the questions that he put to me, I noticed that he wanted to make me feel that he understood me and that I must have patience and trust him. He remained sitting there for another quarter of an hour and then went back to Raf for a bit. I had gone with him to the hallway and saw that now Raf paid no attention to what he said.

He lay curled up in his bed. His eyes were wide open and I saw that he was pretending not to notice that there was someone else in the room. At that Dr. van Thuyl went away again and promised me to come back the next day. When he arrived, Raf again didn't react.

"We must see what can be done to secure admittance for him without his consent," said Dr. van Thuyl. "Raf must be hospitalized, but the question is, how?"

Then he looked at me encouragingly and said, "I'll come again tomorrow to see if I can talk to Raf, although I doubt if it will work. I'll have a think about whether there's another way to go ahead with the admission. I should like his father to be here tomorrow around noon. I'll probably need him."

The next afternoon when the three of us were sitting in the living room, Dr. van Thuyl told us why it was so hard to get a patient into a hospital without his consent.

"Raf is now lying quietly in his bed," he said. "A sectioning order is necessary to authorize me to see to an admission. That's hard to obtain. In Raf's case it must be clearly established that he is no longer in a state to care for himself and that his life is in danger. If you'll help, there's a chance of making this clear to the magistrate. He must, of course, make the final decision. He'll no doubt seek advice from a psychiatrist, but still the grounds must be clear for the magistrate. Therefore Raf will first have to be taken to his house to establish whether he will really starve without help."

I knew that I wouldn't be able to bear Raf

being left all alone in his house in this condition, and we agreed that I would go and stay with my brother for a few days. Dr. van Thuyl thought it best that I left immediately.

"I'll stay with Raf for a little while," Hans said. "And I'll get some food in the house for him."

The psychiatrist arranged with Hans that every day they would go to Raf's house together to see whether he was looking after himself. But it appeared that during their absence Raf hadn't eaten or drunk anything. Furthermore, he showed absolutely no reaction when they came. Hans finally managed to feed him like a little child, but when they came back after two days he hadn't touched any food. When there was still no noticeable change in the situation after a week and Raf was now also talking nonsense, quick action had to be taken to prevent serious danger. Dr. van Thuyl and Hans went to the court, where they were assigned a magistrate who had to grant a sectioning order. The magistrate went with them to Raf's house to be satisfied that there was no alternative.

The admittance to the Bertus Clinic took place the same day.

I felt liberated and all I thought about was a spell of peace and quiet and the possibility that Raf would feel a little better there.

I wanted to hand over my responsibility to somebody else.

Chapter 13 Escape

On my first contact by telephone with the director, I heard that Raf had got medicines that had caused him great agitation. "We couldn't foresee that he would have such a violent reaction to them," he said. "I should like to have a talk with you. I'm not actually treating Raf myself, but as a friend of his father's I still feel responsible for the way things go. I've talked to Raf. Examinations have been done and I've obtained reports."

When I got there he looked serious. "Why have you placed Raf in *our* Clinic?" he asked.

"In the first place, because it was urgent and you could find room for him. But also because Raf has already been in various alternative institutions, and they always had the wrong effect on him. Also, I've read a book by you that gave me confidence in your kind of therapy."

"So what do you expect to happen at our Clinic?"

"In all the years of Raf's illness, I've noticed that he can be helped only with medication, and I was hoping that somebody would manage to get him to take it."

"He hasn't yet refused any medication here," the director said. "But you can't hope for a recovery even with medication. That's why I want to talk to you. Raf is a seriously ill young man, and in the Clinic nothing more can be done for him than to try to make the situation bearable for him. He will most probably even get worse. The clinical picture is unfavourable. Your son is autistic. He has hardly any need for his surroundings. We want to try to stimulate him by finding suitable work for him in the Clinic so that he can still make some kind of contact with other people. How fast this autism will develop further can't be predicted. In spite of all the research, we don't yet know everything about this illness."

"After all these years I understand that very well," I said. "I should like him not to feel too unhappy and not to get into situations through his illness in which there is no way out for him."

It remained a problem to find the right medication for Raf. He was abnormally sensitive to almost everything, thus his muscular movement was so violent that he couldn't get any rest. Within a month he ran away.

I thought that a sectioning order meant that the Clinic looked for a patient who had run away, but that appeared not to be the case. Once again this task was laid on me. They expected me to figure out where Raf was staying. I was told by the Clinic to go to his house to see if he was there. If I should find him, then I was to ring the Area Health Authority, who would take him back to the institution.

I waited until it was evening and then went to see if there was a light on in his house, and there was. I rang up the Area Health Authority and had to take the key of Raf's house to them so that they could pick him up.

But after a few days Raf escaped again, and again I was the one who had to look for him.

Now there was no light burning in his room, which didn't necessarily mean that he wasn't at home. He could be sleeping or sitting in the dark. I didn't dare go into his house, because I realized it was the way I had behaved toward him that was the reason for his breakdown. When I went to look later in the evening, a light was on.

The Area Health Authority thought it was a good idea for me to take them the key again, and once again they picked Raf up. But when within a fortnight he ran away for the third time, I got upset.

The institution did nothing. I, as the mother, had to keep tracking my son down. I rang Raf's psychiatrist from the institution to ask what the point of a sectioning order was if the Clinic kept giving the patient the opportunity to run away. The psychiatrist tried to calm me down.

"We were surprised by Raf's latest escape, too. I had expressly given the order to keep an eye on him. He took a shower in the morning and after an hour he still hadn't appeared. But because we knew that he always stayed in the shower for a long time, they let him get on with it. When a nurse finally went to look, Raf seemed to have disappeared. He had carefully taken all the screws out of the overhead panel of the shower room so that he could work his way through the hole to the outside. I still don't understand how he was able to get out through this small opening."

Again I rang up the Area Health Authority. But the people there had had enough of the whole business, and Mrs. Raas decided that I had to deal with it myself. "I'll have Raf brought back one more time," she said, "but only on the condition that *you* open the door for the A.H.A. male nurses."

"But I can't possibly do that!" I said. "In his eyes that would really mean the greatest betrayal. Raf is already so disappointed in me."

"That's your problem," she replied. "The Area Health Authority will be there. Raf naturally won't open the door if the bell rings. So if you don't let the A.H.A. in, Raf cannot be brought back."

That night I couldn't sleep. I pondered what other alternatives there might be to spare Raf this. When it began to get light I decided to go into his house quietly, in the hope that he would be asleep. Then I would wait in the street for the nurses from the A.H.A. I hoped that *they* would understand the situation and wouldn't force me to open the door for them in sight of Raf.

I tiptoed up the stairs, opened the door, and looked carefully to see if Raf was there. He was sitting on the bed with his clothes on. Tears trickled down his cheeks.

"What is it, Raf?"

He didn't answer.

"Why do you keep running away from there?"

He only said, "Mum, will you stay for a cup of coffee?"

I trembled as I was standing there. How could I go in then? I had come to spy on him and to notify the A.H.A. I said, "No, Raf, I have to go to work," and left quickly.

"Mum!" he called after me. "Mum!"

I didn't dare to look back and disappeared downstairs to wait for the A.H.A. I had no more strength in my legs. My fingers began to tingle. But I had to wait; there was nothing else to do.

After an hour and a half the A.H.A. ambulance came. Raf had fortunately stayed upstairs. I couldn't utter a word. My head felt as if the blood had drained out of it. I handed over the key, tried to say something, but I couldn't get it out. Finally I said with a constricted voice: "Please! Go yourselves."

The male nurse that I spoke to looked at me, took me by my shoulders, and asked worriedly: "Are you OK?"

I just nodded and cried because he understood me.

I was hidden in a doorway when Raf suddenly ran quick as a flash out of his house to the other side of the street. He looked as white as a sheet, paused like a distressed animal unsure which way to turn, and then raced up the street, which in the meantime had filled with people.

I stood with them like an onlooker. I heard them say:

"It's a crazy person!"

"It's a dope addict."

"Look at him go!"

The male nurses went after Raf and tripped him. There was nothing else they could do. They had to get hold of him, and Raf was strong.

I could hardly get my breath and sputtered something out, but little sound came out of my throat. The people looked at me, too, and nudged each other, as if to say, "There's another one."

By this time Raf had scrambled to his feet. His arm was twisted and he was made to bend over like a prisoner. I just looked at his face, of which I knew every feature, and felt my throat constrict.

I ran away from the crowd to a corner of a doorway. Then I began to bawl, with my face hidden in my coat. I felt my arms become leaden. No, not here. I must pull myself together, I thought. I stood there for a long time as though numb. It was hard for me to put one foot in front of the other. My house seemed far away.

When I went into the street again it was oppressively quiet.

Chapter 14   All My Friends Are Crazy

Since then Raf has spent his life in the Bertus Clinic.

In the long run his admission has somewhat relieved the stress. At the time, it was the end of an existence in which he could find no rest anywhere and in which he was dominated by fears and feelings of loneliness, alternating with periods in which he could think lucidly and in which his pain, caused by the realization that he had no further share in the world of other people, became more acute.

During the last two years that he spent in my house, he had suffered more and more because of my distress and my guilt feelings. He keenly sensed every mood of mine, and because of that must have felt increasingly desperate.

My psychiatrist warned me that I should not assume that now nothing else serious could happen. "In psychiatric institutions there are great differences of opinion about policies," he said. "I know that the management of Raf's clinic has to face a lot of problems because of the sensible, realistic approach there. The staff believe in treatment with medicine as the main therapy. They find this the only scientifically responsible approach. Other therapies are also used but only if the patient can handle them mentally. At the moment the Bertus Clinic is still one of the few institutions where they know that seriously disturbed schizophrenics have a right to a home

190

and that this home may also be the institution. Many patients who have been ill for ten to twenty years land in one institution after another – some because the internal policy in their institution has changed, others because their illness has improved temporarily, or because they abscond when their psychotic condition has been made worse for want of sufficient medication.

"It is of the greatest importance for them to be somewhere where they feel at home and aren't yet again told after a while that it's in their own interest to go somewhere else. Some of them are placed in a substitute-family home, where they have to get along with other people much more than they did before and have to live in a smaller space. After they have finally – sometimes after years – felt at home somewhere, they are no longer in a state at an adult age to adjust to so-called family life and comply with the stricter rules of the group. This often goes in tandem with great stress, which can again elicit psychotic behaviour and sometimes serious aggression.

"The upshot of it is – and this certainly applies to schizophrenic patients – that they run away. In the Bertus Clinic they know that for this category of seriously ill people the concept 'hospitalization' doesn't apply. This idea doesn't gain them any thanks. If the prevailing current in psychiatry doesn't want to recognize that people who don't get better also have the right to be cared for, it is very likely that these sick people are going to form a dangerous group of drifters. At the moment Utrecht is made unsafe by a group of neglected, homeless patients whom no institution wants to admit because they need much too intensive treatment. In Italy, too, disturbed people are taken out of old-fashioned institutions. There is great concern about these patients who are neglected and loaf in the streets without being able to look after themselves. All these people are told that society has made them ill. Psychiatry doesn't know what to do with chronic illnesses like schizophrenia, in which there can often be no hope of a recovery. When budgets are cut these people are the first victims, and they are also of no interest to their institution because there's no kudos to be gained from caring for them."

After an exhausting time I got a full report from the psychiatrist about the development of Raf's condition since his arrival in the Clinic. He told me on the telephone that the problems with Raf there were the same ones as in other institutions that he had been in. They wanted to help him but he was apathetic. He had not reacted one whit to his medicines. But they could now say that after three months with much effort they had succeeded after all in making a reasonable beginning with the treatment. Raf was cooperating with them now and they thought they were on the right track.

"In the beginning Raf would sit on the floor for hours," the psychiatrist said. "His long hair hung like a curtain in front of his eyes, so that you could see hardly anything of his face. His appearance got more bizarre by the day. He sat for whole days with his legs right across the floor of the hallway, completely oblivious. His lips moved constantly. He would hold long conversations with himself, in which you would sometimes hear crying and a great deal of sighing. For all that time he held a woollen doll in his arms that he cradled with great tenderness. Later he wore the doll around his neck on a string. Sometimes he would take a diary out of his pocket and write one of his incomprehensible love poems in it. That went on for a month. There was no change. Then we tried another drug, but it made Raf agitated and even aggressive again. Because he kept running away, he himself asked us if he could sleep for a little while in the isolation room. At our wit's end, we also had to discontinue the second drug. Then I gave him something that had been in use for a long time, and its benefit for many patients had already been established."

This medication had an astonishing effect. After just a few days Raf's behaviour changed. The nursing staff had arranged with him that as long as he was so agitated he would do domestic chores. He was happy to do that, because that work tired him out and let him get rid of some of his compulsive movement. After that Raf began to look after himself better, became less apathetic, and sought more connection with other patients. His eyes looked brighter, and he spoke more clearly and stuffed his long hair under his shirt with a scarf wrapped around it. He didn't want it cut, but he also didn't want to shock the others with his hairstyle.

After a few weeks I went to visit him, and I did have to get used to his hairstyle. It looked like an old-fashioned wig.

Raf was still with many seriously disturbed people in the closed section, where people who had just been admitted were observed. But he would soon be transferred to the open section, he said, for he was now getting along well.

The reception room there was very small, so that you sat at one table with other families, and a personal conversation was impossible. It was hard anyway for me to have a sensible conversation when I visited Raf. As a rule I was not relaxed enough and wanted to handle Raf with kid gloves. But now I didn't have to try any more.

Raf had already evidently thought about it and found a solution. He now turned up with a game, so that we could be less tense because we were occupied with something, and now and then we could say something without the painful silence that often fell in these circumstances. This was for me a clear indication of how he had recovered.

He smiled and said, a bit proudly, that he now scrubbed big hallways. "I'm happy that I can do some work here," he said. "I can get along well with the nursing staff and the psychiatrist."

Still, it remained a puzzle to me that he didn't resist when they gave him injections here, while he had refused this in all the previous years.

I had been thinking that he probably understood that he had to accept it because he had been admitted with a sectioning order. But when I was going to have an appointment with the psychiatrist for the first time, Raf said, "Mum, I must warn you, otherwise you won't be prepared. My psychiatrist is a little odd. He has very thin legs and can't walk very well. He undoubtedly once had a serious illness. I think that's why he has a good understanding of other people who are having a rough time, too. I like him. This is something you ought to know."

Maybe that's the reason that he's now accepting medicines, I thought. This psychiatrist had something the matter with him, too.

Knowing Raf, I could imagine that he would have thought: This man is one of us. He's not in perfect shape either, and he'll know what's good for me.

In the meantime Raf was transferred to another section. The visits were tough going there, too. I was often glad when he sometimes took this opportunity to play chess with Hans.

Now he also had a well-defined place in the Clinic. When he had free weekends he rarely came to Amsterdam. He mostly stayed in the vicinity of The Hague and then went into town with fellow patients.

Every two months we spoke with the psychiatrist. He told us that Raf had succeeded in making himself popular with the nursing staff and patients because of the attention he gave to others, even though he still behaved like a loner.

Now that he felt better, he tried to make himself useful in the kitchen when they were washing the dishes. Sometimes he baked cakes for the nursing staff because he enjoyed that work.

Once he brought currants and flour back from the city and made pancakes on Saturday evening for his whole section. This had improved the atmosphere so much that he very often did it.

When I spoke to him about that he smiled and said, "Oh, you used to do that, too. I can't help thinking sometimes now about those days. We enjoyed that, too."

He also liked buying clothing at the market, cheap trousers and shirts. If they didn't fit him, he would ask the nursing staff if one of them wanted to have them. It struck me how well acquainted he was with the current fashion that young people outside the Clinic were wearing. After a year the magistrate, who regularly came to visit Raf, appointed the psychiatrist for the withdrawal of Raf's sectioning order. Raf could now come and go freely, but he did have to abide by the house rules. He had to be present at all the therapy sessions, and there were also domestic chores to do. Raf now followed the rules to the letter.

In spite of all the improvement, I noticed that after a time he withdrew further here, too. As time went on, he stopped going out so often and again also sat staring and talking to himself.

His autism also came to the fore in the Bertus Clinic after around two years, now that he no longer was absorbed by his new surroundings. But he said on one of my visits, "I haven't felt so calm and so well in years. I'm less afraid than I was in those last years at home. It's great that you always have people around you here. You never have to be alone. Sometimes I think that I'd really

196

like to stay here."

The medication also gradually had a negative influence. Raf was, yet again, having more trouble from his compulsive movement, which was sometimes so serious that he couldn't stand still for a moment. When he was calm his gait became more shuffling and his body bent over – the characteristic posture of someone who suffers from autism. He also stuttered badly.

In the therapy sessions he was much occupied with music and during the creative therapy he did a lot of woodcarving, which caught something of his urge to move. He didn't take part in talking therapies. He was present at them because he had to be, but he left as soon as they were over without having said a word.

When they noticed that even in this condition Raf was still in a state to fit into life in the Clinic, they considered letting him live with seven other patients in a little house on the grounds, so that his independence would be encouraged. But Raf chose to stay in the Clinic proper.

In the meantime he had become the manager of the patients' canteen, which during the creative therapy was visited by around a hundred people, and where he had to take care of the coffee and tea and the other details of the organization. They had given him this job so that they could keep him out of his isolation for as long as possible. Up until now none of the patients had stuck with that canteen work for very long. By now Raf had been doing it for a year and the canteen had gradually become an extension of himself.

That was also the reason that he didn't want to leave the Clinic. He finally had a job. He got all his sense of security from it.

Once when I came into his room there was a list lying there of assignments that he had set himself to fulfil.

"It's hard for me to get up early every morning," he said. "But if I don't do it, somebody from the nursing staff comes to tell me that I'm neglecting my duty. Then they nag on and on for so long that it's better to get up right away. There's no getting away from it. They're strict here, and I think that's very good, otherwise a lot of us would just stay in bed. Now I feel just like other ordinary people. I have to."

If you were looking for Raf, you had to look in the canteen first, where he spent many hours.

The psychiatrist didn't like to let Raf out of his sight, and so he hadn't insisted strongly on his going to a halfway house.

When Raf had been in the Clinic for about three years, I noticed that he was cutting himself off from things that happened on the outside. Increasingly, he didn't want to be confronted with them, probably because they could hurt him.

When I came to visit him I had to avoid mentioning any subject that might stir up emotions. I couldn't ask him anything personal and neither could I tell him anything about myself nor about our family. If I did that anyway, he looked at his watch and said that it was time to leave; he had so much to do. I noticed that our conversation went best if I talked about things, not about people. Raf could listen with great interest to travel stories and to stories about my work, but only if these were cheerful. We could also talk about his activities with handicrafts. He felt most at ease if we could take a walk in good weather, because then his compulsive movement had an outlet. He still always found it annoying if Hans or I noticed that he had trouble from side effects. He always remained conscious of his behaviour, I think, and talking about it remained taboo. Once I asked why he had been wearing one glove for more than a month. He looked at me, then at his glove. In fifteen minutes I was standing out in the street.

In the end Raf came to Amsterdam only on birthdays. He hardly ever went to see Hans in The Hague either, although it was nearby, and if he did go he seldom stayed longer than a half hour. Often he left suddenly or unnoticed.

It disturbed us that he cut himself off from us like that and also cancelled our visits more and more often. He kept looking for a reason not to receive me, but on the telephone he would hold long conversations and ask with interest about many things, so that I noticed that he still appreciated the contact.

I phoned the head nurse and asked her if she knew why Raf didn't want me to come and if perhaps something was troubling him that he didn't want to talk about. I asked her whether he perhaps felt unhappy at the moment.

She said, "Mrs. Anstadt, Raf is a seriously ill young man, but he certainly does not feel unhappy here. He empathizes strongly with other people. His family still means a lot to him. Perhaps he wants to protect himself against them, and that's why he reacts that way."

Raf himself said to me: "Mum, will you please ring up when you're going to come so that I'm prepared for it. If you or Dad suddenly appears in front of me, I get an awful shock. My mind goes off on tangents, and then I think that you're somebody else."

Raf has always been aware of his decline, even now. He has been in the Clinic for four years now.

The last time that he came to visit me on my birthday he was remarkably quiet and stared into space with a sad smile. Through this quietness from time to time disconnected thoughts occurred to him, which seemed to arise out of long pondering.

"I feel very old," he said. "As old as you are."

"I have nothing more to look for in the city."

"My former friends and I have nothing more to say to each other."

"I enjoy the Clinic most of all. I'm going back."

"I know hardly anybody here any more."

"All my friends are crazy."

.